"But My Doctor
Never Told Me That!"

*Secrets For Creating
Lifelong Health*

Contact Information:

Judith Boice, N.D., L. Ac.
11520 SE Main St.
Portland, Oregon 97216

Phone: 877–5BE–WELL
(877–523–9355)

website: www.drjudithboice.com
e-mail: drjudith@drjudithboice.com

"But My Doctor Never Told Me That!"

SECRETS FOR CREATING LIFELONG HEALTH

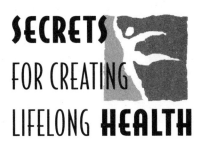

Judith Boice N.D., L.Ac.

ALTHEA PRESS
11520 SE Main St.
Portland, OR 97216

Althea Press
©1999 by Judith Boice N.D., L.Ac.
All rights reserved. Published 1999
Protected under the Berne Convention

Cover by Marcy Rouske
Design by Carolyn Riege
Illustrations by Maya Andrea Y. Grillo Massar
Printed in the United States of America

08 07 06 05 04 03 02 01 00 99   5 4 3 2 1
ISBN: 0-9670453-1-2 (paperback)

The publishers have generously given permission to use extended quotations from the following copyrighted works. From *How Shall I Live*, by Richard Moss, M.D. Copyright 1985 by Richard Moss, M.D. Reprinted by permission of Celestial Arts, Berkeley, California. From *Power Sleep*, by James Maas, Ph.D. Copyright 1998 by James B. Maas, Ph.D. Reprinted by permission of Random House, Inc. From *Creating*, by Robert Fritz. Copyright 1991 by Robert Fritz. Reprinted by permission of the author. From *Your Money Or Your Life*, by Joe Dominguez and Vicki Robin. Copyright 1992 by Vicki Robin and Joe Dominguez. Reprinted by permission of Penguin Books, Inc.

Note to reader: The information in this book is in no way intended as a substitute for medical counseling. Please do not attempt self-treatment of a medical problem without consulting a qualified health practitioner.

ACKNOWLEDGEMENTS

For several years I have been exploring how to meld the process of creating with the world of healthcare. The work and teaching of Robert and Rosalind Fritz inspired this exploration, and without them this book never would have come into being. I am deeply indebted to Robert Fritz for his genius in clarifying and teaching the creative process. This book is my humble attempt at applying Robert's teachings to the world of health care, offering a fundamentally different approach that focuses on creating health rather than avoiding symptoms or preventing disease. Rosalind Fritz gave invaluable feedback on the manuscript. Her insights challenged me to further refine the ideas presented in the book. Thank you both – you are greatly honored teachers and mentors in my life.

Special thanks go to Ann and Gary Ralston who helped guide the creation of this book as well as my long-term visions. You have been wise counselors and unwavering coaches. You speak the truth without flinching. Thanks, I needed that!

Thank you, Dr. Lynda Falkenstein, for providing invaluable coaching throughout the creation of this book. I appreciated your careful, insightful comments and your uncanny ability to define and woo the market place.

Thank you, Mom and Dad, for financial and moral support while I devoted myself to writing the book. I am deeply grateful for your ongoing love and support. Mom, you have an extraordinary ability to hunt down the precise spelling and correct grammar in the most obscure cases. You win my Grammar Cop and Spelling Queen awards hands down!

Elizabeth Robinson, thank you for the copy-editing expertise and an unprecedented number of belly-laughs. I've never had so much fun getting feedback from an editor.

Thanks to those who read and commented on the manuscript. Your thoughts and reflections helped refine the manuscript. Thanks to William and Martha Boice, Brooke Ann Lyon Burnett, Dr. Libby Guimont, Regina Kerr, Dr. Rick Kirschner, Ann Ralston, and Kiji and Lolita Watters.

I am especially indebted to the wonderful artists who designed various aspects of the book: Marcy Rouske, cover; Carolyn Riege, design; and Maya Andrea Y. Grillo Massar, illustrations.

To my sister Ruth (1957 – 1998),
with thanks for your encouragement
in writing this book.

Contents

Chapter 1.
Dale's Story   1

Chapter 2.
Secrets for Optimizing Health   25

Chapter 3.
The Oracle of Hygieia:
Secrets for Creating Lifelong Health   81

Chapter 4.
Secrets For Nourishing Your Body   115

Chapter 5.
Classified Information About Exercise   171

Chapter 6.
Secrets Your Doctor Never Told You
About Mental/Emotional Health   197

Appendix A   237

Appendix B   240
Journey to Health Chart
Diet and Exercise Journals
Exercise Questionnaire

Endnotes   250

CHAPTER 1

Dale's Story

Dale arrived for his 1 P.M. appointment looking relaxed and confident, moving like a well-oiled athlete. At 48 years, he worked as a forester and took pride in his physical condition. He ate a very healthy diet and ran five or six miles every other day. He possessed a spiritual understanding of the world that provided a sense of joy in his life. Despite his age, he had a boyish sense of mischief about him. As a friend, I knew him to be a Pied Piper among children, one who enchanted with his stories and endeared with his untiring sense of fun. He also shared his deep reverence for life through the sweat lodges he led at the turn of the seasons. For him, The High Level Wellness Program©, as he said later, ". . . looked like a cake walk."

The previous autumn Dale's wife Paula had completed the Wellness Program, and he arrived that late January afternoon for his history and physical with some knowledge of the program. He brought his completed goals and values worksheet, diet diary, exercise journal, and *Stress Map*. After reviewing the information he had collected, we added to the already extensive medical history he provided. His only complaint was a recent decrease in endurance. He couldn't keep up with the younger foresters playing basketball the previous summer, and he noticed the crew had to wait for him when walking up steep hills. He attributed these changes to his reduced exercise program in the past year and reported he had started running again this autumn. He mentioned pain under his right shoulder that was better with exercise and after lying down. Over the last four months, the pain had started progressively earlier and earlier in the day. Dale had no other health concerns.

Far from being a devotee of doctors of any stripe, Dale had not had a complete physical exam in 25 years. We began the exam, quickly moving through fingernail and lymph node inspection and then examining eyes, ears, nose, and throat. I listened to Dale's lungs with a stethoscope and then moved my hand over his chest to check the heart. I could feel his heart beating through his chest wall, no matter where I placed my hand on his chest. I quietly reported the finding to my team member, third year medical student Valerie Simonsen, who was charting the findings. I continued the exam, punctuated with quiet notations.

"PMI [point of maximum impact] laterally displaced." Pause. (Normally you can feel the heartbeat most distinctly just below the nipple. Dale's PMI was farther to the side.)

"Blowing murmur between S1 and S2, loudest at the fifth intercostal space. I'd say Grade 3." (If the heart is healthy, you cannot hear murmurs.) Pause.

"Abdominal aorta, four to five centimeters wide."
(Normally about two centimeters wide.)

On visual inspection, Dale's rib cage shook with each heart beat, even while lying on his back. I turned to meet Valerie's eyes, wondering if she recognized the import of the findings. Her furrowed eyebrows reflected her understanding. Dale lay quietly on the exam table, eyes closed, breathing deeply. The verbal chart notes had not interrupted his relaxation.

I completed the exam: no water retention in the legs or abdomen, and no carotid bruits or reduced pulses in the feet, all possible signs of congestive heart failure. "Dale, you can continue relaxing while I check on some things. We'll be back in a few minutes."

We spent the rest of the afternoon trying to contact Kaiser Permanente, Dale's Health Maintenance Organization (HMO). Initially his primary physician refused to talk with us, certain that a "naturopath" would have no credible medical findings to report. We requested he make an appointment for Dale with a Kaiser cardiologist. The physician refused, suggesting instead that "if he continues to have problems," Dale report to the emergency room at Kaiser.

We performed an EKG in the clinic, and then Dale and I discussed future testing at Kaiser. We reviewed a drawing of the heart and discussed how the heart compensates for a valve disorder.

I knew we needed more testing to make a final diagnosis, and I pleaded with Dale to stop running until we had completed the evaluations.

"But I feel great," countered Dale. "Why should I stop running?"

"I would feel much better if you walked until we have all of the testing done. You can walk briskly, but running may not be such a good idea right now." I hesitated to tell him my greatest concern – that, in addition to the valve disorder, he might be developing an abdominal aneurysm (weakened and enlarged blood vessel) as well.

Still unconvinced about abandoning his running schedule, Dale left the clinic with instructions to visit Kaiser for a chest x-ray and echo-cardiogram.

Dale's cardiologist joins the team

I talked with Dale the following day after reviewing the EKG, which indicated enlargement of the left side of the heart. Dale had visited the emergency room at Kaiser (he couldn't make an appointment with a cardiologist for weeks), and reported that after the initial screening tests the emergency room nurse had the same recommendation: "Please walk, don't run, until we have completed all of the testing." After the second plea, Dale was willing to adopt a walking program.

Dr. Aaron Angel, Dale's cardiologist at Kaiser, consented to have me accompany Dale and his wife Paula on their first office visit. After listening to Dale's heart and reviewing family and past medical history, Dr. Angel leaned back with one arm folded over his

What this means for you:

Have annual exams. You can decide what to do with the results of the exam. At least you have information to make choices!

4

chest, the other thoughtfully curled over his upper lip. "The echo-cardiogram shows an aortic prolapse — the valve is not shutting all the way. That's why the heart has enlarged, to compensate for the 'leak.' You probably will need a valve replacement, but before we jump to that conclusion, we need to check some other things, like making sure the coronary arteries are not blocked, which I think probably is not a problem at your age, with your background."

My mind raced through familiar territory. Dale and I had already discussed valve replacement, the types of valves available, and the probable sequence of events if he chose not to have an artificial valve surgically implanted. "Your physical abilities will decrease over time," I had told Dale, "usually starting with difficulty shoveling snow, then mowing the grass, later climbing stairs, getting into the bathtub . . . ."

"That's where I stop," said Dale, halting the list of progressively restricted physical activity. "At that point, I check out."

I had nodded quietly, knowing that Dale was struggling with the idea of any sort of intervention, surgical or otherwise, to sustain his health. I knew that after a very full and physically active life, Dale would find the steadily diminishing range of physical activity intolerable. He was jammed between a rock and a hard place – in this case, an ideological dilemma and an unacceptable physical reality.

The new feature in the terrain I had not expected was the location of the valve disorder. From the position of the murmur when listening to the heart, I had assumed a dysfunction of the mitral valve (the valve opening into the left side of the heart), and was surprised to hear the diagnosis of aortic valve regurgitation (blood sloshing back into the heart through an incompletely closed valve). In my mind, the landscape shifted, revealing a much more serious condition. Because the aortic valve is the gateway between the heart and general circulation, the aortic valve labors under the highest pressure of any valve in the heart. A diseased or damaged aortic valve can cause complications in the heart, lungs, and general circulation as well.

"The next step," continued Dr. Angel, "is an angiogram. That's a procedure where we make a small incision in the femoral artery, in the groin area, and insert a catheter – a tube – to inject dye into the heart. The dye allows us to visualize the blood flow in the heart and in the coronary arteries. You generally feel a sensation when the dye is released in the heart. Most people describe it like a rush of warmth from their toes up to their head. It doesn't last long. The whole procedure usually lasts about an hour. Any questions?"

Dr. Angel answered Dale and his wife's questions, mainly about the need for medication following valve surgery. Dale would have to take Coumadin, a blood thinner, for the rest of his life. Coumadin would reduce the risk of clot formation caused by the mechanical valve.

A nurse escorted us into a room to watch a video about the angiogram procedure. A moderately overweight, middle aged man described his progressively worsening heart symptoms and the doctor's decision to order an angiogram to evaluate the condition of his coronary arteries. The video followed him through surgery prep, the procedure itself, and then back to his lakefront home where he and his family were enjoying a picnic complete with steaks and potato salad. The treatment for his coronary artery disease obviously did not include dietary recommendations. Overall, the video gave a very complete, reassuring description of the angiogram procedure.

Food for the body and the spirit

On Dale's next visit to the clinic, we discussed dietary recommendations, in this case a soup-only diet designed to minimize the work of his digestive system and maximize the absorption of nutrients. The diet was meant to reduce the load on his cardiovascular system and prepare his body for the anticipated surgery. We discussed the vitamins and minerals, botanicals and homeopathic remedies that would help prepare his body for surgery. We also checked his Chinese pulses, three positions on each wrist, and gave an interpretation of how the pulses reflected his organ functions.

Dale drew in a deep breath and met my eyes. "You know, I thought this program would address the spiritual side of things. I'm just getting more information about all the things that are wrong with my body."

Dale was naming my worst fear, that western medical

training had crowded out my spiritual understanding of the nature of our bodies. Had the medical system remolded me and crippled my understanding of the wholeness of life? I was barely breathing, waiting for him to finish.

"Instead of feeling good when I leave this clinic, I leave feeling like there's something else wrong with me."

"Dale, I'm sorry you feel that way," I said, trying not to sound defensive. "The reality is that something is malfunctioning in your body right now, but that's not the whole of your body. I hate being the bearer of bad news, but I can't ignore what's going on. I would be irresponsible if I overlooked the condition of your heart. I'll do my best to keep what's going on with your heart in perspective. You do have a very strong, resilient body that has compensated beautifully, for a long time."

We sat silently for a few moments, eyes locked. "I'll do what I can to focus more on the spiritual aspect," I said quietly, "and I need to bring up the physical side as well."

I felt awful for most of that week, wondering if I had failed my patient miserably. At the peak of my distress, I called Dr. Caroline Myss, a friend who works with intuitive diagnosis. She is an inspired source of clear reflection and wise counsel. The clarity of her reflections is not always pleasant for me, and I awaited her comments with nervous anticipation.

After outlining the basics of the case and my own

self-doubt about my interactions with Dale, she halted my litany of self-reproach.

"Look," said Caroline, "you saved his ass, and he's ungrateful. You don't need to apologize about what you're doing. I refuse to deal with people like that, who want to blame me for their diagnosis."

"Well, I don't think that's what he's doing . . . ."

"You don't have to apologize, sweetie. You did the right thing."

I felt relieved when I hung up the phone, free of an enormous burden. I realized that I was struggling with the line between listening empathetically and absorbing responsibility for a patient's distress. How could I listen to someone's distress, especially when aimed at me, and not take the issues personally? I also needed an internal barometer to gauge when criticism was justified, requiring a change of behavior.

After the telephone conversation, I began to realize that Dale's reaction probably reflected a natural cycle of grieving – first denial (he rarely talked about his heart condition outside of office visits), then anger, followed by bargaining ("If I do this, Creator, will you give me that?"), depression, and finally acceptance. I sensed that Dale was progressing through the initial stages of grieving.

Caring for the Earth, tending the body

During our next office visit, we discussed exercise changes, searching for ways to bring more enjoyment to Dale's walking program. He loved running and was making peace with substituting walking as aerobic exercise. We talked about ways of bringing a meditative focus to his daily walks, using the exercise as a way of increasing his body awareness. Dale already practiced yoga and did relaxation exercises.

Slowly the conversation shifted to the topic of surgery, and the possibility of a valve replacement. Dale strongly believed in allowing the body to function without artificial intervention and already had legal papers declaring that no artificial life support was to be used in his medical care.

We talked about a concept introduced earlier in the Wellness program, that our bodies are microcosms of the planetary body. "My body, my flesh and bones, are the part of the Earth that I'm most directly responsible for," I commented. "Taking care of this body automatically links me with caring for the Earth. And sometimes, just like the Earth needs intervention to clean up a polluted or damaged area, my body needs intervention to rebalance it, too."

I don't recall much of the specifics of the conversation, but I knew I was direct and caring, having abandoned my self-doubt earlier in the week. Later in the day, when all the Wellness Program participants met for our support group session, Dale surprised us with a decision he had made that afternoon.

"I've spent my life committed to caring for the Earth," he began, "and I've been thinking a lot about that commitment this afternoon . . . . Something happened today, and I realized that I am committed to taking care of my body, just as I'm committed to taking care of the Earth. I decided to go ahead with the surgery. And my reminder of that commitment to my body will be the [Coumadin] pill I will have to take every day."

Tests and trials

Two weeks after the first visit with Dr. Angel, Dale checked into Kaiser for angiogram surgery. With Dr. Angel's generous consent, I observed the procedure. Dale looked relaxed and calm before surgery. He chose to receive only local anesthetic during the procedure, bypassing the offer of muscle relaxants and painkillers to ease the discomfort of lying on the flat, hard gurney for the duration of the surgery.

The surgical part of the angiogram usually lasts about 10 minutes, but we were in surgery for almost three hours. Dale received more unexpected news. The initial part of the procedure went as expected. The first dye injection, recorded on video as an x-ray in motion, revealed turbulent flow in the left ventricular chamber. The second step was to insert the head of the catheter into one of the coronary arteries. The catheter generally bends at the correct length and angle for insertion into the artery, but in Dale's case the catheter did not come close to reaching the opening. A slow but steady flow of other cardiologists and lab technicians entered the surgical area, offering advice on catheter sizes and rereading the x-ray studies.

Dale endured, tolerating the procedure beautifully, until he glanced at the video monitor and connected the image of the catheter moving through blood vessels with his own body. His heart rate dropped to 40 beats per minute as the shock registered in his mind. Dr. Angel injected atropine to restore a normal cardiac rate, and then morphine to reduce the discomfort of the prolonged procedure.

At the end of the morning, we had more information about the condition of Dale's heart. The catheter did not fit at the correct angle in Dale's heart because his aorta was enlarged, skewing the usual angle of insertion. Dale had an aortic aneurysm, subject to burst at any time. If the aortic wall did give way, the internal blood loss would be rapid and fatal. After having made the difficult decision to proceed with surgery, the cardiologist was unsure that Dale's heart was repairable.

"When doctors spend a lot of time with you . . ."

Dale and his wife spent the next day discussing what they would do if Dale died. In shock myself, I talked with Dale later in the day.

"I'm learning something," reported Dale.

"What's that?" I asked.

"When doctors spend a lot of time with you, it's a bad sign."

I laughed. "I guess you're right. Otherwise, they're on to the next patient."

"I was telling Paula that in the High Level Wellness

Program one of the questions they ask is 'What would you do if you had six months to live?'" Dale paused, chuckling. "I told Paula I'm in the advanced Wellness Program. In the advanced Program they tell you you have six months to live – now what do you want to do?" We both laughed.

We talked about how he felt about dying, and any unfinished business he might have. "Well, actually," said Dale, pausing a moment, "I'm kind of curious about dying, about what comes next. I've never died before. It sounds kind of exciting to me."

"You're amazing, Dale," I said, shaking my head against the telephone receiver. "That's a great way to look at death."

Dale already had traveled to California to tell his son Jeremy about his heart condition, and he had arranged visits with his parents and other family members. He and Paula planned outings, including a visit to the beach where they had gone on one of their first dates. They were making peace with living life fully, as long as life might last.

Two weeks later, Dale completed a treadmill cardio-vascular evaluation to rule out any blockages of his coronary arteries, a substitution for the angiogram view of the arteries. Dale also had MRI (Magnetic Resonance Imaging) testing of his chest region. After the tests, he went to see the surgeon who would perform the operation.

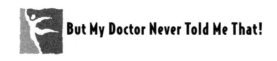

Dale's surgeon joins the team

Dr. Ahmed listened to Dale's heart and then reviewed the MRI films with us. Dr. Ahmed escorted Dale and me into his consulting room to discuss the required surgery – reinforcement of the aortic wall as well as replacement of the aortic valve. During the visit, I outlined Dale's pre-surgery protocol with Dr. Ahmed and asked if he had any modifications or additions to recommend. After answering his questions, we discussed the alarming increase in the cancer patients he saw, especially younger people, and escalating environmental toxicity in the U.S. Dr. Ahmed also inquired about a naturopathic physician's scope of practice. He seemed genuinely interested in my responses.

Although Dale was ready to proceed immediately with surgery, Dr. Ahmed wanted to wait three weeks, until the beginning of April, when a new prosthetic material would be available. This improved Dacron material would stabilize the aortic aneurysm.

Prompted by Valerie's request, I asked Dr. Ahmed whether Valerie and I could observe the surgery. I assumed that the operating room had observation windows. I never would have asked had I known that we would need to be in the operating room (O.R.) Dr. Ahmed readily consented, but his nursing staff vehemently protested. They did not want any potential distractions during a long and complicated surgery. The nurses finally relented, agreeing to a brief observation period during surgery.

Gazing into the heart of life

Dale continued the pre-surgery protocol and soup-only diet. He and Paula hosted a steady stream of friends and family members. "I didn't know so many people cared about me," commented Dale. Toward the end of the three-week wait, though, Dale grew tired of retelling his story and weary of the constant reminder of what lay ahead. His brother's family arrived from Alaska, and they escaped for a magical week of camping along the California coast. When Dale checked into the hospital the afternoon before surgery, the ocean was only one day behind him. He was bronzed and relaxed. Several staff members asked him what he was in for. He certainly did not look like a typical cardiac patient.

The morning of surgery, Valerie and I arrived at the hospital at 7:00 A.M. and spent about an hour visiting with Paula and her sister in a beautiful waiting area created for families of patients in cardiac surgery. Diana, a nurse at the hospital and good friend of Dale and Paula, joined us at the end of her night shift. Paula settled in for a long vigil.

Around 8:15 A.M. the head surgical nurse escorted Valerie and me into the locker room and showed us where the scrubs were kept. We donned shirts and pants, slippers and hair nets before entering the hallway leading into the operating theaters.

We greeted Dr. Ahmed who explained the surgery preparation had been prolonged because Dale's core body temperature had to be lowered slowly, over an hour's period of time, before the surgery could begin. The reduced temperature would help minimize the effects of the long surgery. Dale's chest was open, and Dr. Ahmed wanted us to see the size and condition of the heart and aorta. Afterward, they would perform the bypass that would shunt blood from the right atrium into a machine that oxygenates the blood; then they could begin the repair of the aorta and left ventricle.

Valerie and I followed the nurse into the operating room, quietly waiting in the corner for the crew to acknowledge our entrance. "Everyone has their own way of dealing with the tension," whispered the nurse. "This is a particularly complicated surgery, so the tension is really high. They'll let us know when they're ready for us."

After a few moments, the anesthesiologist motioned us forward to a stool placed directly behind Dale's head. The anesthesiologist spends most of the surgery perched right above the patient, ready to alter medications almost instantaneously if needed. For a few moments, though, she relinquished her position, and Valerie and I took turns standing on the stool, looking down into Dale's pulsating heart.

I'm not exactly sure what I expected. I had spent most of the night in semi-sleep, roused often by a restless sense of expectation. Only two years before I had cried after drawing someone's blood, certain that I was inflicting horrific pain. Never would I have imagined that I would walk through that fear and pain to stand in this spot, witnessing a major surgery.

Instead of fear or pain, I was overcome with a deep sense of wonder as I gazed into the mystery of a living, pulsating body. The heart was enlarged, the aorta the size of a goose's egg, but the wholeness of the heart and its rhythmic beauty overwhelmed me. I was looking into the very core of the mystery of human life.

The nurse escorted us to another operating theater. "Dr. Ahmed wants you to see what a relatively normal sized heart looks like." Again we took turns standing behind the patient, gazing into the core of the body, observing the ebb and flow of life.

The journey home

Dale emerged from surgery seven hours later. At every stage of his recovery, Dale's body responded beyond everyone's expectations. Before midnight, the nurse removed his breathing tube. The day after surgery he was sitting up eating lunch. Within three days he left St. Vincent's and was transferred to Kaiser's hospital. On Sunday morning, five days after surgery and five days earlier than expected, he returned home to complete his healing process.

The journey of recovery did have some unexpected turns, however. Twice Dale experienced episodes of numbness in his arms and was rushed back to the hospital. Both times the EKG showed no abnormalities, and after a night of observation, Dale returned home. Less dramatic but equally important were the biweekly blood draws to evaluate his clotting time. Some of the supplements we had prescribed to speed Dale's recovery from surgery were on a list of restricted substances because of their effects on clotting time. I spent a morning researching drug-supplement interactions and discovered several mechanisms that would account for a decrease or increase in clotting time. A literature search of journal articles over the past five years provided very little information. Presumably interactions between drugs and supplements are low priority when allocating research dollars.

The nurse at the coagulation clinic could not explain any mechanisms for the drug-supplement interactions, but she did report observed changes. More than 1000 mg of vitamin C, for example, would speed the clotting time. My research suggested that vitamin C speeds clotting time because it catalyzes the pathway in the liver that breaks down Coumadin. Less drug in the system means increased tendency for blood clotting. We were learning that the smallest changes in diet, supplements, or lifestyle could significantly effect Dale's clotting time. Dale had acquired a feedback system that quickly reflected the effects of his lifestyle on his body, via the changes in his clotting time.

Surgery – the double-edged sword

The experience of working with Dale taught me a great deal about working with someone during a major life transition. Human interaction, especially during a time of crisis, transforms the world of medicine from a science to an art. The Chinese character for "crisis" is a combination of the characters for "danger" and "opportunity." Surgical intervention presents a double-edged sword, with the dual possibility of leading into or out of danger. Faced with the option of a slow, degenerative disease that would hamper his physical abilities or the dangers of a major surgery, I believe Dale chose wisely. Of course that conclusion is easy to reach in retrospect, with the outcome a certainty. If Dale had died on the operating table, I'm not sure how I would view his choice. He would have avoided the misery of a slow demise but lost the experiences, the suns and moons and sorrows of the last years of his life.

Developing a collaborative relationship with your physician(s)

Dale's experience illustrates the importance of including the patient in the healing team. Dale participated in his "program" from start to finish. His feedback, challenges, questions, and most of all his decisions greatly affected his health. I gave Dale all the information, support, and feedback that I could. Ultimately the decisions were his – whether he would endure tests, have surgery, follow treatment recommendations, etc. We actively exchanged feedback about what was or wasn't working for us, as doctor and as patient. Together we shared a common goal: Dale's vision for his health. We had that final desired outcome against which to measure the success of our work together.

In addition to Dale's vitality, humor, and courage, I believe his successful recovery was due at least in part to the cooperation of his physicians. After the surgery Dr. Angel, Dale's cardiologist, commented that my work with Dale was remarkable for three reasons:

"First, because you went into the O.R.," explained Dr. Angel. "I've never been in the O.R. Most surgeons wouldn't even let their mother in the O.R. to observe a surgery. Second, you followed Dale through the entire process [from diagnosis through treatment]. And third, during the cardiac conference following the surgery, Dr. Ahmed was praising your pre-surgery protocol. That's unheard of."

Dale succeeded in drawing together a health care team that was "remarkable" on several counts, demonstrating that medical professionals from diverse backgrounds can work with one another to serve a patient's best interest, while in the process drawing forth each other's strengths and special skills.

My experience with Dr. Angel and Dr. Ahmed confirmed my belief that physicians can work together harmoniously for the benefit of the patient. This experience led me to expand the High Level Wellness Program to include a core of health care practitioners from many disciplines. In such a setting, everyone benefits from the wisdom and skill of several medical orientations, presented within a coordinated health care program.

How to use this book

I chose to begin this book with Dale's story to provide an example of the workings of the Wellness Program in a real life situation. Using this volume as a guidebook, you can follow the same basic framework as High Level Wellness Program participants.

- *The program began with a thorough evaluation of Dale's lifestyle as well as a complete medical history and physical exam.* I highly recommend you have a complete physical before you make any major lifestyle changes. Complete the questionnaires and journals on pages 100-105 of Chapter 3 to generate an accurate "snap shot" of your current lifestyle.

- *Dale attended lectures and participated in weekly support groups.* The information presented in each chapter covers most of the material presented during the lectures. I have tried to make the information as "user friendly" as possible, to approximate a knee-to-knee conversation. The book, however, cannot substitute for a support group. You may choose to read the book with a group of friends and meet after reading each chapter to share your challenges and successes. In the program, the support group has three ground rules: 1. Make "I" statements (I speak about my own experience, not assuming "We all _____ " or "You all _____ "). 2. Whoever is speaking has the floor (no interruptions or cross-talk). 3. Meetings begin and end on time.

- *We tailored the three major sectors of the program (nutrition, exercise, and mental/emotional health) according to Dale's particular needs, in this case preparing him for surgery and then supporting him in his recovery. Other patients had different recommendations, based on their particular needs and challenges.* Work with your doctor(s) to customize the information presented in the nutrition, exercise, and mental/emotional health chapters. See Appendix B for more resources to help you fine tune your lifestyle choices.

- Some people can master several lifestyle changes at once. Others may need a slower, steadier approach. If you are in the latter group, give yourself at least two weeks to integrate the information in one chapter before moving on to the next.

- You may choose to photocopy the forms in the appendix so you can reuse them in the future.

- This book can never take the place of a health care provider. Ideally you would be working with a physician who is experienced in making lifestyle changes. If your doctor is unfamiliar with this approach, gently educate her. Offer information. Relay your experiences, both the successes and the mishaps. Eventually your physician may choose to seek this information as well, especially if you and others are demanding such care.

The journey of a lifetime . . . .

The secrets contained in this volume are meant to assist you in creating lifelong health. The changes you will make and the benefits you will receive are part of the larger journey of your life. We will be discussing lots of details along the way, but keep the landscape in mind. Set your sights, lace up your boots, and prepare for the journey of a lifetime.

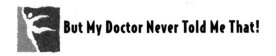 **But My Doctor Never Told Me That!**

NOTES:

CHAPTER 2

Secrets
for Optimizing
Health

During the summer before my third year in medical school, I began to ask myself questions about wellness. What factors contributed to or undermined health? If I really wanted to focus on optimal health, what kind of practice did I want to create, and how did I want to spend the next two years of my clinical training? I was on a plane flying cross-country after a visit with family and friends on the East coast. At the beginning of the flight, I knew only that I was not particularly interested in spending the majority of my time treating acute conditions like indigestion and earaches. I knew what I didn't want, not what I wanted.

During the flight I reviewed the journey that had brought me to "classical" medicine, the ways of healing that pre-date our conventional medical system. I grew up completely dependent on the conventional medical system. Beginning at six weeks old, I was sick with alarming regularity. Before I was a year old, my mother summoned the doctor for a late night house call, fearful that a high fever would consume me. The doctor faithfully prescribed antibiotics for each round of ear infections, colds, and bronchitis. The physician did not understand that antibiotics destroy health-promoting as well as disease-causing bacteria, making the body more prone to future infections. At eight I endured a staph infection in my lower intestine that went undiagnosed for several months because the doctor assumed that I "didn't want to go to school" and was feigning illness. At nine I was hospitalized with pneumonia. At twelve, I suffered with phlebitis. These frequent early childhood illnesses taught me about pain, drug reactions, and the debilitating effects of repeated antibiotic prescriptions. Finally, when I was 13 years old, my mother's persistent demand for an answer to my chronic upper respiratory infections paid off. "She exercises and eats a healthy diet," my mother told the doctor. "Why is she always getting sick?"

Our family doctor referred me to an eye, ear, nose and throat specialist who had me tested for food allergies. I was allergic to many of the "healthy" foods I was eating. Perhaps those foods were nourishing for other people, but not for me. Within a couple of weeks of eliminating my food allergens, a three-month bout of bronchitis cleared. Avoiding a relatively long list of food allergens seemed a bargain compared to the cost of chronic illness. I happily avoided the foods, found more nourishing substitutes, and began reading everything I could find on nutrition, exercise, and overall health. I knew I had reached the end of what the conventional medical world had to offer. Within another year I was jogging almost daily, taking a multi-vitamin and mineral supplement, and eating a diet that was healthy for me.

> **SECRET #1:**
> **Begin where you are.**

Already sick and tired of being sick and tired
at age 13, I had to rebuild my health from a badly
compromised foundation. I had to start where I was –
exhausted and demoralized, with a debilitated immune
system and a wrecked digestive tract from all of the
prescription drugs I had taken. I had to regain strength
before I was able to exercise. First I made the dietary
changes, added supplements, and then started an
exercise program as my energy increased.

I have observed a similar pattern among patients
who seek classical medical care. Either they have
reached the end of the world they know, having exhausted the offerings of conventional medicine, or they
are motivated to improve their health. One group
is running desperately from the ravages of chronic
illness, the other toward a vision of greater health.
In either case, classical medicine requires something
that conventional medicine does not – participation.

> **SECRET #2:**
> **You can learn to create health.**

Conventional medicine views the body as a car
and the doctor as a mechanic who can fix the ailing auto.
In this car-mechanic model, a patient has little responsibility for the "repair" work other than swallowing the
required pills or showing up for a scheduled surgery.

The patient does not change the structure of her life to support health, but rather depends on the physician to discover the magic bullet that will eliminate discomfort. Wielding no magic bullets, and at best devoid even of the concept of an arsenal, classical medicine offers the gift of education, guiding people to live in a way that supports their innate health and vitality. Natural therapeutics help to correct imbalances, and at times serve to reduce pain and other symptoms. These palliative interventions support patients until they are able to make the broader, more far-reaching changes that ultimately will restore their health.

Secrets for creating lifelong health

Most of my academic and clinical education prepared me for the business of prescribing medicines that would rebalance the body and reduce pain, but very little of the training prepared me for the art of assisting people in making lifestyle changes that ultimately would support their health. I knew that my passion was to work with people in the midst of life transformations who wanted to construct the foundations of health.

During the remainder of the flight, I wrote about the "basics" of a healthy lifestyle. The foundations of health include nutrition, exercise, and mental/emotional health. The recipe for a complete, health-sustaining lifestyle required all three of these basic ingredients.

How could I create a program to assist people in

realizing their health goals? To be successful, I knew that a program would have to incorporate the following secrets for creating lifelong health:

SECRET #3:
Create your own personal definition of health.

Develop a picture of yourself in perfect health that is detailed enough that you will recognize "health" when you achieve it. More detail does not necessarily mean a greater chance of succeeding. Have just enough detail to identify accurately when you have achieved your goal. If your doctor or someone else provides the inspiration for making changes, what will you do when you the program ends or your "motivator" moves out of town?

SECRET #4:
Make changes for a lifetime.

If you lose 50 pounds for your 20th high school reunion, will you maintain your weight when the party is over? If you choose to sustain a healthy weight for the rest of your life, you will probably maintain the weight loss. If your commitment ends when the dance floor lights fade, you probably will regain the weight and more after the reunion.

> ### SECRET #5:
> ### Participate in your health care.

Learn what you need to know to achieve your health goals and then maintain them. You don't necessarily need to know everything, just the information that will move you toward your goal.

> ### SECRET #6:
> ### Seek individualized health care.

Many "wellness" programs are one-size-fits-all constructs that ignore the individuality of the patient. Certain information does apply to everyone, e.g. basic nutritional requirements or the elements of an exercise program. The application, however, varies widely according to a myriad of other factors such as fitness level, physiological needs, and life situation. One person, for example, may thrive on a fruit-only diet in the morning, while someone else with low blood sugar may need complex carbohydrates or proteins for breakfast. Work with a physician who focuses on lifestyle changes who also knows when to recommend supplements, pharmaceutical drugs, or surgery. As we saw in Dale's story, some people do need drugs and surgery to correct extreme conditions. Drugs and surgery alone, however, cannot produce vibrant health.

This book is a journey, an odyssey intended to support you in the creation of lifelong health. Initially we will focus on your vision of health – what does health look like for you? Do you want to be healthy for a lifetime? We will explore these questions in Chapter 3. In this chapter we will delve into a system of medicine that augments health rather than simply eradicating symptoms. After all, if you eliminate a symptom (or a problem), what are you left with? You have the absence of the problem, not the creation of something new. Rather than focusing on how to eliminate symptoms, I would encourage you to ask yourself, "What does health mean for me? What do I want to create?"

The most lucrative investment of all

Most westerners do not invest in health. We tend to seek immediate gratification of our desires and focus a blind eye on the consequences of our actions. Recently during a lecture tour I had a long discussion with the owner of the bed and breakfast where my colleague and I were staying. The innkeeper asked what naturopathic medicine could do for diabetes and high blood pressure. We discussed diet and exercise changes that can completely eliminate the need for insulin or oral medications. We reviewed the long-term risks of unchecked diabetes: blindness, systemic infections, kidney failure, and loss of lower limbs. He was well versed in the long-term effects of the disease.

31

"Well, I know I should be doing other things," he said, affectionately eyeing the Famous Amos chocolate chip cookies crammed in cookie jars throughout the house. "I just can't give up my sweets. I mean, I grew up cooking, and I love to cook. How could I give that up?"

"Who said you have to give up cooking?" I asked. "You may just need to change the focus on what you're cooking . . . ."

"Oh, but I love the creamy gravies, the desserts, the waffles and pancakes with syrup in the morning, all of that stuff . . . and besides, I'm cooking for the guests here, too."

We talked more about the pharmaceutical industry. He had worked for several years as a representative for one of the major pharmaceutical companies, and he had many war stories to recount.

"I'm amazed," I told him, "at how many patients would rather take a pill, and live with the side effects, than make some simple changes in their lives. The pharmaceutical companies thrive on the myth that drugs can save us from ourselves, from the poor choices we make that damage our bodies and destroy our health."

"Right," muttered the innkeeper, "like me and my cookies." He also mentioned a television commercial aired earlier that evening that promised amnesty from gastritis if the advertised pill was taken before indulging in some indigestible gastronomical bomb. Pills to prevent discomfort – paying the Piper before he's even piped!

Unfortunately, the commercial forgot to mention

that eventually we do pay for our indulgences, for the "withdrawals" we make from our bank account marked "health." Eventually we overspend, exhaust the account, and operate on "credit" – energy borrowed from coffee and other stimulants, drugs, alcohol, sugar, etc.

The next morning, as we were preparing to leave, the innkeeper finally felt comfortable enough to ask his most pressing question: "Do you know of any cures for impotence? Have you worked with anyone with impotence?"

"Yes, I have," I told him. "The cure depends on the cause of the impotence. If someone is impotent from taking high blood pressure pills, there's really nothing he can do other than get off the pills. That goes back to making the lifestyle changes that would allow someone to discontinue the medication."

"Right," he said, looking defeated. "The pill can't take away the high blood pressure without some side effects. There really is no substitute for making the changes, is there?"

"Unfortunately not if you want to be healthy."

I wrote this section before the introduction of Viagra, currently the most lucrative drug in the pharmaceutical industry. Originally developed to dilate blood vessels for the treatment of heart disease, pharmaceutical companies quickly recognized a more profitable use for the drug – the treatment of impotence. Many men refused to take medication for high blood pressure when they realized the drugs blocked their ability to have an erection. Now the pharmaceutical companies can cash in twice – increasing blood pressure medication sales and their new wonder drug to deal with the side effects of the first prescription.

Choose your health investments wisely. Putting life energy directly into a healthy lifestyle often yields a far greater return than the money spent on pharmaceutical drugs. Taking one drug usually leads to taking several others (to treat the side effects of the first drug). Investing in one health supporting activity (e.g. exercise) often leads to gains in other healthful activities (e.g. eating better and sleeping more). Whatever you invest in grows, so plant your seeds with care.

How much do you value your health?

Zig Ziegler, a motivational speaker, asks his audience if they would spend millions of dollars on a race horse and then let it stay up late watching movies, drinking beer, and eating Twinkies. The audience laughs at the ridiculous picture, yet many of us treat ourselves with similar disregard every day. We value the health of the animals in our care more than we do our own.

What this means for you:
Compare how much you spend each year on alcohol, movies, cigarettes, and/or junk food with how much you spend on healthcare. Your cash flow provides clues about what you value most.

Why do you want to be healthy?

Dr. Willis Harmann of the Noetic Sciences Institute has been studying cultural trends for the past two decades. Remembering that any system of categorization has its faults as well as its strengths, Harmann's system can not completely explain our motivations for the choices we make, but his findings make some important distinctions. Initially he found that most people's source of motivation fell into one of three distinct categories: survival-directed, outer-directed, and inner-directed. To illustrate these different motivations, imagine why someone might want to lose weight.

The survivalist would choose to lose weight because his girth somehow threatens his survival: "I have to lose weight or I'll have to buy a whole new closet full of clothes, and I certainly can't afford that." The survival-oriented person maintains the same perspective no matter how much or how little money is in his bank account. Even millionaires may be survival oriented.

The outer-directed woman would choose to lose weight so she would look good, or so she looked as good as someone else. "Oh, I have to lose ten pounds to fit in this year's bikini style. I'm planning to go to the Bahamas. You know, that's the 'in' place to be this year! *Vogue* magazine says so, and I want to look good in my new bathing suit. You-know-who just might be there . . . ."

The inner-directed man makes choices based on his own values and desires. He may choose to lose weight because he notices he has more energy when he is ten pounds lighter. He may decide he wants to improve his health by losing weight. He is moving toward his goal, rather than flogging himself with survival fears or "motivating" himself based on the opinions of his neighbors. He generates choices internally.

The survival- and outer-directed people most likely will forget their decision to lose weight. As soon as another pressing issue threatens their survival, or another fashion makes a splash, these people will shift their focus away from their desire to lose weight. Usually inner-directed people will complete their goal, in large part because their motivation is not dependent on external circumstances.

We will discuss the importance of goals and desires more in the next chapter.

What this means for you:

Why do you want to be healthy?

What is your vision for your life?

Your health?

The secrets of classical medicine

While developing a definition of wellness for yourself, you may want to consider some of the following principles that guide the practice of classical medicine. Throughout this book the term "classical" denotes medical systems that predate our contemporary conventional medical system, which relies chiefly on pharmaceutical drugs and surgery for its "cures." Most of the conventional medical profession focuses on helping patients move from a lying to a sitting or standing position. Once upright, or "functional," the patient is on her own to further improve health. "Classical" medical systems also can assist in moving from a lying to a sitting or standing position. In addition, classical medical systems offer ways to move from standing to walking, possibly even dancing, in our physical forms.

Classical medicine has roots that go back to classical Greek times, and that reach even deeper into earlier ages when healers drew medical knowledge directly from Earth wisdom. Examples of classical medical systems include Ayurvedic, Naturopathic, and Traditional Chinese Medicine. Folk herbal traditions also stem from the same roots. The following maxims derive from the philosophy of naturopathic medicine, yet they would apply equally well to any classical medical system.

SECRET #7:
Work with the body's innate ability to heal.

Both our human bodies and the Earth have an innate wisdom that governs the cycles of birth, growth, maturation, and decay. We humans are microcosms of the planetary condition, and our strength lies in aligning ourselves with the universal principles that support life and health.

Instead of supporting the body's ability to heal, most pharmaceutical drugs attempt to suppress symptoms. In other words, most prescription drugs sweep the garbage under the rug instead of moving the trash out of the house and dumping or recycling it.

Corticosteroids, for example, reduce inflammation,

irritation, and swelling by disabling the immune cells that trigger inflammation. With long term use, corticosteroids cripple the immune system and destroy connective tissue, e.g. skin, bones, and muscles. Corticosteroids push exterior symptoms deeper into the body. Applying hydrocortisone cream on an eczema outbreak behind the knee, for example, may resolve the irritation and itching. Once the rash has disappeared, however, the person often develops asthma. The hydrocortisone cream has swept the symptom "under the rug," deeper into the body, in this case from the surface skin into the lungs. Interestingly, when the asthma resolves, the eczema often reappears. The body finally

What this means for you:

Pharmaceutical drugs cover symptoms; they do not resolve the cause of the symptoms.

has gathered the strength to push the disturbance back to the surface. Unfortunately, when the eczema reappears, most people apply hydrocortisone cream again and once again push the disturbance deeper into the body. This cycle of treating eczema with corticiosteroids and then suffering with asthma may repeat again and again until the person finds a way of addressing the root of the problem – the underlying allergic tendency that makes him or her prone to develop eczema, asthma, and/or hayfever.

Earth wisdom, body wisdom

Our human bodies are wise, imbued with the ability to adjust to innumerable moment-by-moment shifts and changes. The Earth, too, has a finely tuned system of checks and balances. NASA hired British scientist James Lovelock, author of *The Gaia Hypothesis*, to create a definition for "life" that could be used in assessing the presence or absence of life on other planets. Lovelock decided to use the Earth as an example of an "alive" planet. In his research he discovered that the Earth functions as a self-regulating organism, just as our own human bodies do. The salinity of the ocean, for example, has remained constant for several million years. By laws of physics, the oceans long ago should have become far too salty to support any life form. Similarly, the percentages of atmospheric gases have remained constant for billions of years despite great fluctuations on the planet's surface. The Earth becomes polluted or diseased only when these compensatory mechanisms are overtaxed.

Like the planetary body, our own human bodies have an intrinsic imprint of balance, a "set-point" that serves as a template for health. Without this internal knowledge, the organism cannot respond appropriately to external or internal changes. In a balanced system, the set point generates appropriate "cravings" that support health. Infants and young children whose tastes have not been skewed by highly processed foods usually gravitate toward foods that support their growing bodies. Humans and other animals naturally draw inward when they are hurt or ill. The organism understands the need to rest, to lie still, so that the body may devote its energy to regeneration rather than movement or digestion.

When out of balance, the body craves substances or environments that further undermine health. When protein-deficient, for example, we crave chocolate and refined carbohydrates. Alcoholism and low blood sugar are linked in a chicken-or-egg syndrome – alcoholism may cause or be caused by low blood sugar problems. We often develop cravings for substances that cause allergic reactions. The "rush" generated by the body's immune and glandular systems can become addictive. The ensuing "crash" when the body recovers from the hormonal surge leads to a desire to take/eat/smoke/drink the substance again for the initial jolt it produces. The crave-consume-high-crash-burn-crave cycle can be very difficult to break once the system is off balance.

A time for healing

Engaging the body's natural healing abilities requires making time an ally. Many western pharmaceutical drugs excuse us from being rooted in the cycles of time. "But I don't have time to be ill," says an exasperated patient. "I have so many things to do. I can't just stop everything and be sick!"

Having become accustomed to the lightening-speed effects of potent drugs, we have a distorted idea of the time scale required for natural cycles of healing. Ironically, too, the drugs may disrupt the body's ability to respond to imbalances and create more disease. Often the medicine the body most desperately wants is time. Illness provides an opportunity to stop, reflect, rest, and reconnect with healthier rhythms. Those who over-step this process are vulnerable to repeated illnesses until they reestablish those rhythms. An herbalist, instructing me in how long to follow a treatment plan to address a particular illness, suggested I devote a month of herbal treatment for each year the patient had suffered with the disease. A month? I said to myself at the time. In retrospect, though, the exchange of a month of treatment for a year of illness is a bargain. Our bodies are temporal organisms and must be rooted in the cycles of Earth time and seasons if they are to maintain physical balance.

> What this means for you:
>
> *Take time to rest! Often the most potent treatment for colds and other acute illnesses is sleep. Some people need as much as 9 or 10 hours of sleep to maintain health.*

The human body also can be damaged to the point of losing its ability to rebalance on its own. Infusions of love, care, attention, and appropriate supportive treatment can return our bodies to health much more quickly than if left to falter on their own. "Natural healing" means more than simply leaving something alone to take care of itself. The laissez faire method will work if the body is not too badly damaged. Severe damage, however, requires skillful, supportive intervention to rebuild a healthy body.

Elements as allies

Many of the means to rebalance the body derive from natural elements: earth, air, fire, and water. Earth, for example, heals in the form of clay and mineral nutrients. Fire has been used for centuries to induce an artificial fever, e.g. a sauna or sweat lodge, to cleanse the body. Clean air and appropriate breathing techniques nourish the body with oxygen. "Hydrotherapy" includes many different types of treatments, all involving applications of hot and/or cold water. As well as describing our internal healing abilities, the "healing power of nature" also refers to the therapies derived directly from the Earth's elements. The elements' native, "natural" intelligence interacts with our own bodies' healing wisdom to bring about balance, harmony, and health.

Life cycles

We humans participate in cycles of growth and maturation, death and decay, just as all living organisms on this planet, and the Earth itself, wheel through cyclical patterns, with each stage providing the foundation for the next. Infants, for example, must experience crawling before walking in order to support normal physical and mental development. First a baby crawls unilaterally, moving the right foot and right arm forward at the same time. In the second stage of crawling, the baby "cross-crawls," moving the right arm and left leg, then left arm and right leg. In addition to developing physical coordination, cross-crawling helps synchronize the two halves of the brain. Without cross-crawl stimulation, the baby bypasses an important developmental stage.

At the completion of our life cycle, death is part of the natural cycle that precedes rebirth. I give away my body so that other beings may use the elements of my physical form to create the structure of their own bodies. The molecule of water "dies" from river to grass, from sedge to foraging insect, from grasshopper to bird, from robin to hawk, from predator to the watery arteries of the Earth once again.

For a culture that so celebrates the "paradise" promised in heaven, I am puzzled by the fear of death in our culture. If the spirit exits the body for some celestial resort, then why do we invest in caskets for our loved ones that are air-tight to slow the process of decomposition? Do we secretly hope to preserve the body in case the heavenly resort is booked up, or worse yet, closed?

Some cultures understand life fully enough to practice the art of dying. I treasure the few examples I have of people who inhabit their lives so completely that they make their deaths an act of grace. Scott Nearing, author with Helen Nearing of *Living the Good Life* and numerous other books, was inspired both in his living and his passing. On Scott's 100th birthday many friends and neighbors gathered at the Nearings' home in Maine for a parade and celebration. Shortly afterward Scott told Helen he thought 100 years was "enough," and he was ready to go. He began a juice fast, then after a couple of weeks took only water. On his last day, he lay in bed with Helen sitting at his side. They expressed their love and said, "Goodbye." When he was ready, Scott closed his eyes, took a deep breath, and died. Peacefully. With grace. He was a masterful practitioner of the art of dying.

What this means for you:

Take time to notice and celebrate major life transitions.

In our headlong rush to "get on with our lives," we often miss the depth and wisdom of these transformational times.

Our bodies are infinitely flexible organisms that are designed to live and move in graceful balance. The Earth body and our human bodies are infused with a wisdom that maintains this elegant balance. This wisdom, or "healing power," underlies the principles of health that govern life on this planet. To live with these principles is to strengthen the innate processes of life; to defy the wisdom of the body is to create separation from ourselves, and ultimately the Earth. To fully inhabit the planet, we must first inhabit our own physical bodies, rooting in the flesh and bone of earthly experience. This wisdom, or "healing power," underlies the laws of health that govern life on this planet. Our union with earthly rhythms ultimately links us to the greater cosmos. We become earth-bound stars dancing to a celestial music, enmeshed in the larger patterns of life.

SECRET #8:
Notice how your life affects your health.

Illness does not occur without cause. The body, in its elegant wisdom, always whispers before it shouts. Improve your health by learning to listen to your body and its early warning signs. Body symptoms are metaphors, or perhaps more accurately markers, of shifts and changes in our lives.

Roots and branches

Treating the cause means addressing the roots of an illness, not the stems and leaves that symbolize signs and symptoms in the body. Several diseased roots may lead to the manifestation of one symptom, or damage to one root may cause several withered branches on the tree. "Bugs" will not invade a tree unless the vital force of the organism has been weakened.

The same is true in our bodies. Infections cannot "take root" in our bodies unless our bodies are weakened, e.g. by extreme environmental conditions, stress, lack of nourishment, or emotional upsets. Chinese medicine refers to the treatment principles of *Ben* and *Biao*, the roots and the branches of disease. The skillful physician learns to differentiate between deep-seated causes (Roots) and the symptoms (Branches) of illness. Treating the branches of an illness only has a short term effect, while addressing the roots offers the possibility of "cure," by re-establishing a healthy foundation. Of course, the roots and branches are related – in combination with the trunk, they form the body of the tree. Carefully observing the Branches helps us trace back to the Root in order to treat the cause of a disease.

Ancestral inheritance

Unlike most Westerners, Chinese medicinal practitioners view our genetic inheritance as mutable, capable of change over time. The Chinese rule of thumb is that a "genetic" disease requires seven generations of healthy living to clear it from one's genetic or ancestral memory. Within this framework, a healthy lifestyle not only benefits health and well being in this lifetime, but also provides the foundation for the generations that will follow. In a sense we leave an inheritance of good health for future generations.

What this means for you:

The better the parents' health at the time of conception, the bigger the health "bank account" their child inherits.

Classical medicine also recognizes the importance of the parents' health in determining a child's well being. In essence, the foundation of the child's health can be no stronger than the combined strength of the parents' health at the time of conception. Couples interested in conceiving a child are encouraged to commit a full year to building both the father's and mother's health so the child has the largest "bank account" possible from which to draw at the time of conception. The Chinese call that fixed amount of life force available at birth "Jing," an energetic substance that functions like the pilot light on a stove, providing the ongoing spark that maintains the flame of life.

Energetic causes of disease

Our bodies respond not only to physical elements but also to the more subtle energetic realms that provide the "juice" or "qi" [chee] that sustains our lives. Without this enlivening force, our bodies would be nothing more than sacks of bones and fluids. Many cultures have developed health practices that cultivate the life force or "spirit" that informs our physical bodies. One such practice is Qi gong [chee gong], a Chinese method of using mind, breath, and body to restore health.

Exhausted after months of non-stop traveling and teaching, I was desperate last autumn to find a way of refilling my depleted body and spirit. Through a series of events, I returned to the oriental medical school where I had earned my degree to study with Professor Chen, a Qi gong teacher with a remarkable history. Chen's suffering began in childhood with severe digestive problems. During her adult years she also struggled with crippling arthritis and daily migraine headaches. Finally, at age 49 a doctor diagnosed Chen with terminal cancer and told her family she had only two months to live. Rather than giving her a prognosis, the doctor advised Chen to "go home and rest, eat lots of good food, and relax," which was the doctor's gentle way of saying, "We can do nothing for you. Go home and die."

One day while waiting for radiation therapy, Chen chatted with the man beside her. He, too, had been diagnosed with terminal cancer. He listened, smiling, while Chen recounted her lifelong struggles with illness. His smile never faltered. "I began to wonder if there was something wrong with him," says Chen, laughing.

When she finished her story, the man beside her recounted his own diagnosis of terminal cancer and his quest for a "miracle" cure. He had searched throughout the city and finally discovered a group of people in a park doing slow-motion exercises – Qi gong. He watched, fascinated, and eventually joined the group. Many were cancer survivors who attributed their recovery to the effects of Qi gong.

Chen joined the group but initially felt none of the energetic sensations other long-term practitioners described. "I didn't feel any of that at first," she explains, "but I knew it was working because I began to feel better. My health improved. That's how I knew it was working." Now, 16 years later at age 65, she maintains a busy teaching schedule, guiding others in the practice of Qi gong. Always smiling, moving lightly, she easily could be mistaken for a much younger woman.

How can a set of slow motion exercises cure the body of cancer? The purpose of the exercises is to use mind, breath, and body to move qi (life force) and blood throughout the body. The practice also increases vital energy in the body. When we accumulate enough vital energy, diseases can no longer take root in the body. As the cells literally begin to vibrate at a faster frequency, cancer and other diseases cannot survive at the new energetic level.

Who are we, then, if our bodies are little more than shifting molecules of vibratory matter? Our bodies are complex expressions of genetic as well as vibratory information. The cause of disease can be pursued right down to the level of quantum physics – the electron, the flash-in-a-pan micron of energy, whose position or speed, but never both, can be tracked at one time. Pursuing final causes leads us inevitably back to the realm of energetic medicine. In restoring health, our job is to match the information from the vibratory realm with practical applications in the physical world. "Cosmic," energetic information means nothing if it cannot be applied in the day-to-day world of our waking lives.

Rather than initiating a desperate search for an energetic explanation for illness, I hope these ideas encourage you to consider the impact of energetic therapies in healing the body. Only in the past few decades have Western scientists begun to explore the more subtle energetic patterns in the body. We have learned to measure gross electrical patterns, e.g. using the electrocardiogram (EKG) and electroencephalogram (EEG) to measure electrical activity in the heart and brain. We have been slow to conduct more subtle explorations in part because we do not have good tools to measure energetic phenomena. Our inability to verify the effects of electrical, magnetic, and other energetic influences on the body probably has more to do with our primitive tools than the validity of the healing methods. Piling rocks on one end of a see-saw while the patient sits on the other end of the see-saw, for example, is a very primitive way of measuring weight: Mr. Smith weighs 1 boulder, 2 rocks, and 17 pebbles. Many of our energetic measuring tools are equally primitive. Thankfully, other cultures have explored these energetic realms with tools and devices acceptable in their own cultural context. We in the West are beginning to understand mechanistically what other cultures have known through other means for centuries. Stay tuned. We will continue this exploration of the causes of disease in Chapter 6.

The most popular (western) way to die

Today's most common cause of death in the U.S. and most industrialized countries is coronary artery disease. Chinese medicine offers insight into our cultural tendency for heart disease. Keep in mind that Chinese medicine describes the body more poetically than does western medicine. The Chinese developed their medical understandings from thousands of years of careful observation, not dissection or double-blinded experi-

W h a t t h i s
m e a n s f o r
y o u :

Vibrant health

requires more than

good food, exer-

cise, and supple-

ments. Discover

your own way of

nourishing your

spirit, e.g. yoga,

Qi gong, cere-

monies and

celebrations,

prayer, meditation,

music, and/or time

spent in wilderness.

ments. From the Chinese medical perspective, both joy and sadness affect the heart. Watch someone with advanced heart disease for any length of time, and you will see that they quickly shift from tears to laughter, back and forth, like flames rising and receding from dying embers. The Chinese associate the heart with the element of fire, our source of warmth and vitality. Fire can also burn out of control, destroying all in its path in a fiery burst of energy.

The power of fire is tempered with water, an element controlled by the kidneys. If the kidneys are depleted, they cannot perform their nourishing and cooling functions. The heart's fire burns out of control, manifesting in heart disease including hypertension, arteriosclerosis, and heart attack.

The Chinese have learned over the millennia how to nourish and support the kidneys. During the winter season, associated with kidneys and water, the Chinese pay special attention to nourishing this vital organ. They rest more, allow time for the dreamy winter darkness to nourish their watery natures, and eat foods and drink teas that warm and nourish the kidneys. The Chinese understand the principle of storing energy for the future, living in a way that increases their vital strength so that it can be used when needed in the future. The kidneys are like the body's energy bank account, and they make regular deposits in that energy storehouse.

Our western culture has no concept of storing energy for the future. During most of our lives we are spending our life energy. Often by the time we reach middle age, we have depleted the bank account and are operating on "credit," energy borrowed from stimulants such as coffee, black tea, diet pills, and drugs. We live on debt, borrowing energy and thus health from our future. If we become too overdrawn, our life force dwindles, sometimes to the point that any deposit of care and attention, no matter how great, cannot balance the deficit. Too late we begin to eat properly, rest, exercise, practice stress reduction, and attempt to open our hearts to love. Without the ongoing nourishment of water, the fire burns too hot and consumes the remaining vitality of the body.

Water is also associated with the emotions. Over the last three decades many in our culture have learned to feel and express emotions. The men's movement, encouraging men to feel and express the full range of their emotions, may well diminish the prevalence of heart disease in current medical practice. Already researchers have found that " . . . inexplicably, death from coronary heart disease has declined in the United States since the late 1960s."[1] Perhaps the emotional opening of the last three decades is in part responsible for the decrease in heart disease in our culture.

A study designed by Dr. Dean Ornish demonstrated that changes in diet and exercise combined with emotional work can reverse coronary blockage. Emotionally opening the heart correlates with physically opening the blood vessels that nourish the heart.[2] Obviously emotional expression is not the only factor implicated in lowering the incidence of heart disease, and Ornish acknowledges that all lifestyle factors (diet, exercise, emotional balance, and stress reduction) contribute to coronary health. Many physicians, however, overlook the importance of stress and emotions in treating heart disease.

I offer this example of heart disease as an exploration of the root of an illness. Usually many factors contribute to the development of an illness. I do not subscribe to a theological view that illness is a punishment for sins or wrong doing, nor the laissez faire attitude of accepting suffering as a natural part of living. The New Age doctrine espouses a world that is "perfect," in which we unequivocally create everything that befalls us. Illness, in truth, is unpredictable, often mysterious, neither positive nor negative. The cause is usually multi-faceted and unique for each individual.

Symptomatic treatment

Cutting at the branches of a diseased tree is like treating the symptoms of an illness. We see immediate results – the reduction of a fever, the elimination of skin infection – but the underlying cause of the imbalance still festers in the roots of the organism. In fact, symptomatic treatment suppresses the disease and drives it deeper into the body. When the disease is virulent, we may need to treat both the *Ben* and the *Biao*, the roots and the leaves, but the skillful physician always returns to focus on the roots of the disease when the acute episode has passed.

The creation of health depends upon a lifestyle that supports the integrity of the organism, that fertilizes the roots with appropriate nutrients so that the body can skillfully rebalance itself. Rather than heroically slashing at diseased branches, we can learn to nourish our tree of life so that it may bear fruit for ours and future generations.

What this means for you:

If you have a recurrent symptom or condition, you probably have been treating the branches and not the root. Once the root is healed, the branches return to health.

SECRET #9:
Choose the least invasive treatment possible.

As we noted earlier, the body whispers before it shouts. In treating the body, I prefer to nudge the body gently before strong-arming it with invasive, potentially destructive therapies. The more invasive therapies sometimes work more quickly, but what do we "pay" for the quick fixes of conventional medicine? Some of us pay with our lives.

A *Journal of the American Medical Association* (JAMA) study demonstrated that appropriately prescribed drugs, both prescriptions and over-the-counter (OTC), account for over 100,000 deaths annually. In addition, 2.1 million people each year are "injured" as a result of pharmaceutical prescriptions. Legal prescriptions and over-the-counter (OTC) drugs are the sixth leading cause of death in the United States.[3]

Classical, natural therapeutics aim to rebalance the body with the least invasive treatments possible. In practice, a classical practitioner begins with the simplest treatments (e.g. dietary changes or hydrotherapy) before adding more complex, and often more expensive, treatments. I would rather nourish the body to support the body in healing itself before choosing treatments that "attack" a symptom directly. I also aim for the simplest, most effective treatment – elegant simplicity. I will prescribe a single, well-balanced formula before recommending a bagful of supplements.

"Doing no harm" also includes implementing therapies that nourish and strengthen the body. Conventional medicine has few if any drugs that support the body. The majority of the pharmaceutical arsenal is aimed at destroying things in the body. In contrast, both western and eastern classical medical traditions employ "tonics," herbs and other formulas that strengthen the body. These tonics generally are prescribed after long term illnesses, after births (for the mother), and for preventative care. The Chinese, for example, often drink special teas and eat certain foods at the change of each season to prepare the body for new environmental conditions. Until the 1950s, the U.S. Pharmacopoeia included several tonifying herbal formulas, often referrred to as "spring tonics." In the past half-century, we have almost completely lost this medical understanding of rebuilding and strengthening the body. Often when I mention tonics in public lectures, people stop me, curious to know what I am talking about. Thankfully we are relearning the wisdom of regenerating the body through nourishment and tonification.

Naturopathic tradition adds the understanding that digestion must be improved in order to optimize the absorption of healthy food. The most lovingly cooked food gathered from a local, organic garden will benefit the body only if the digestive tract can break down and absorb the food. Many classical medical practitioners prescribe digestive tonics to improve the flow of gastric juices and promote the healing of an inflamed or damaged intestinal lining.

The Chinese tradition includes the use of tonics to strengthen organ systems as well as the intangible "Wei Qi" [way chee] that defends the body against disease. The tonifying herbs alone, however, cannot heal the person. Diet, exercise, and relaxation also play a vital role.

A word of caution: tonics strengthen all aspects of the body, including invading diseases. Taking a tonic during a cold or the flu may actually intensify and lengthen the illness. Sometimes tonifying herbs are added at the end of a long, debilitating illness. Consult a well-trained Chinese herbalist before taking a tonifying remedy while you are sick.

What this means for you:

Tonics rebuild and strengthen the body. Use only while healthy or during recovery, NOT during the acute phase of an illness.

56

Choosing conventional medicine

For some patients, especially those who have waited until their condition has progressed far into the realm of pathology or who were diagnosed late in the disease process, drugs and surgery may be valid options. I have observed people who were so determined to avoid any sort of technological medicine that they rejected the most appropriate treatment for their condition and for themselves as human beings.

Richard Moss, M.D., relates the story of a patient whom he counseled regarding a benign tumor in his middle ear. Actually, Moss simply listened to the man, not only to his words but also to the energy and feeling the words conveyed. The man was certain that the best way to work with the tumor was to "heal himself." Over a period of visits, though, the man began to realize that surgery might be a doorway, leading him to equal or greater fulfillment than his intended "spiritual" approach. According to Moss,

> I saw that the deepest aliveness didn't make distinctions between [conventional] medicine and holistic treatment or between daily life and spiritual life. The [conventional] medical or surgical procedure is as much a part of the mystery of life as anything else and is a true door to wholeness. In its present form, it is also a new door, one that is here because of the way we live today. We are always trying to get rid of threatening doors: grief, uncertainty, pain, death, disease. Often we succeed. But a life

without doors is too one-dimensional to encompass
the depth and mystery of aliveness. . . . The German
mystic poet Rilke regarded modern man as a dark
fortress, the windows shuttered, the drawbridge
pulled up. To this image he whispers, "Don't you
sometimes wish for the enemy?" The "enemy" is
any experience that has the capacity to let in the
light and open us to the mystery of life. In such an
experience, we have to acknowledge, finally, that we
don't know anything, that we never did, and that we
are not in control. Being out of control is unbearably
frightening for most of us; we are forever protecting
ourselves. Doors were needed in the past as they
are today and the way through is the same then
as now.[4]

The tools of conventional medicine are not
inherently "evil," certainly not to be avoided at all costs.
Like any tools, they can be used to build or destroy.
Perhaps the most dangerous aspect of the conventional
medical paradigm is the way in which the practitioner
views the patient – uninformed, powerless, obedient and
childlike, respectful of the greater knowledge amassed
by the Scientific Doctor/God. The doctor also suffers in
this paradigm. Patients expect practitioners to diagnose
and treat correctly 100 percent of the time. They expect
brilliant, painless treatment plans from physicians who
have only two cannons at their disposal – drugs and
surgery. Patients expect to be "fixed," no matter how
advanced the disease, no matter how great their neglect

in caring for their own bodies.

I am deeply grateful for the gifts of pharmaceutical drugs and surgery. When used properly, these technologies can correct very serious conditions. Physicians and patients can collaborate, working respectfully with each other to implement these tools. Certainly Dale, my beloved friend, would not be here today without the miracles of open-heart surgery and Coumadin.

Restoring Natural Rhythms

During the late autumn, when the Oregon sky dims to a gray, half-lit glower, I find myself retreating inward, almost grateful when the pale sun dips below the horizon and the blanket of night rests upon the land. Like the deciduous trees that have released their leaves and drawn the sap into their core, I too find myself energetically contracting, focusing my attention inward, irresistibly drawn into dreamy contemplation. Over the years I have discovered that honoring this inward pull builds a steady strength that resists the seasonal plague of colds and the flu as well as the emotional "blues" (the color associated with Kidney) that often accompany the holiday season.

The body, as a microcosm of the Earth, responds with varying energetic patterns during the annual cycle of the seasons. In spring, the body vibrates with an abundance

> **What this means for you:**
>
> *Drugs and surgery are not inherently evil – in some instances they save lives. Conventional medicine, however, can be misused, such as taking pre-scription antibiotics for a viral upper respiratory infection.*

of energy, beautifully matched with the explosion of light and life that greets the season. Winter plumped bodies become firm tending the garden, mowing grass, and walking on the vernal green belly of the Earth. The body moves into a steady, active state during the summer in tandem with the ripening, maturing flora and fauna of the land. In autumn, the body begins to turn inward, slowing as the light decreases and the days grow colder. Activities become more mental and less physical as the cycle moves into the stark inward season of winter.

Our body also honors daily patterns, in a sense mimicking the yearly seasonal cycles within the context of a single rotation of the Earth. We move through periods of activity, reflection, and rest, which follow the ebb and flow of cortisol and other hormones in the blood stream. Often in our western culture, we overlook the need for reflection and rest. Electric lights burning long after the departure of the sun are metaphors for the condition. We live as if the sun were always up, ignoring the power of night and its dreamy, restive gifts.

"Natural" cravings?

Although I would like to offer blanket approval for following what appear to be body "instincts," I am aware that our bodies develop "cravings" that are an outgrowth of unbalanced lifestyles. The body may cry for sugary foods when the underlying need is increased protein or magnesium in the diet. The craving for sugar, in this case, is a perverted attempt to restore balance in the body. One of the side effects of over-riding body wisdom for any period of time is that the body develops cravings that, ironically, do not support body health. Instincts arise from a balanced state; cravings result from imbalance.

Restoration Ecology

Perhaps the gentlest, most effective way of restoring order in the body is to focus on areas of strength. The concept is both obvious and revolutionary. Most medical practices focus on what is wrong with the body and overlook the myriad systems and processes that continue to function beautifully.

The field of restoration ecology applies this understanding to the healing of environmental systems. A restoration ecologist begins by acknowledging points of strength and then discovers ways of protecting those areas so they can flourish and eventually spread to encompass surrounding "diseased" areas.

While living in Scotland I witnessed the principles of restoration ecology being applied to the regeneration of the native Caledonian forests. Vast forests once covered Scotland, ranging over 1,500,000 hectares of mountainous land. Today only 12,500 hectares of scattered forest remnants remain, less than two percent of the original Great Forest. The heather covered mountainsides are

---

What this means for you:

Sorry, a PMS-fueled kamikaze mission for chocolate is not a healthy instinct, but rather a craving that provides clues about nutritional imbalances. Chocolate cravings may result from a magnesium deficiency, while sugar cravings may signal a lack of protein and/or the mineral chromium.

---

not a natural phenomena, but rather the land's second growth attempt to cover the denuded slopes bereft of trees. Walking through the heather moors, one can still find stumps of Caledonian pines, the tenacious roots remarkably well preserved in the boggy soil.

In response to this situation, Alan Watson initiated an innovative program called "Trees For Life" to regenerate the Caledonian forests. "A basic principle of restoration ecology," explains Watson, "is to begin from areas where there is still greater biological diversity and fragments of the ecosystem to be restored." The restoration of Highland glens includes not only the regeneration of Caledonian pine trees but also oak, birch, aspen, alder, rowan, juniper trees, and many species of moss and fungi. Restoration efforts also encompass reintroducing native animals that once roamed the Caledonian forests: wild boar, brown bear, elk, reindeer, and wolf.

A major challenge threatening regrowth of the forest is overpopulation of deer and sheep. In the last 20 years, the Highland deer have increased from 200,000 to 300,000 due to a series of mild winters and an increase in shelter provided by commercial monoculture forests. The deer also lack natural predators to curb their population – gone are the wolf, brown bear, and wild cat.

Trees For Life builds fences to protect forest remnants from grazing deer and sheep. The forest responds to this protection with an extraordinary show of vigor, with young tree seedlings growing at an exponentially speeded rate. Over time the fences are extended to protect larger tracts of land. The vitality of the fenced areas also seems to have spilled over into the surrounding hillsides. Seedlings within a half-mile of the fenced enclosure have escaped from the grazing deer, struggled beyond bonsai stage, and grown to a size that defied the grazing animals. The concentrated efforts aimed at regenerating the fenced areas have also affected the surrounding moors.

Like the beleaguered forests, our bodies can also benefit from the principles of restoration ecology: protect what is healthy, nurture what is strong, and over time extend the aegis to include more and more of the body.

Remember the power of simple things

When restoring health, look first for simple treatments. Often simple remedies are dismissed as powerless or useless, which is an understandable perception when they are compared with the cannon-like instruments of the pharmaceutical armamentarium. Some ailments, however, require nudges, not nuclear weaponry. Why shove the body when gentle encouragement will suffice? Why choose drugs with a foot-long list of side effects when dietary changes or an exercise program will accomplish the same goal? In some cases, someone may need drugs and/or surgery. In such cases, classical medicine can often combine with conventional medicine to help reduce trauma and speed recovery time. The classical practitioner aims to restore and nourish, to persuade rather than pound the body. Depending on the severity of the illness, the body will often respond with a surprisingly minimal intervention.

> **SECRET #10:**
> **Develop a collaborative relationship**
> **with your physician.**

The word "doctor" derives from the Latin word *docere*, meaning "to teach." A classical physician functions primarily as a teacher, providing information and coaching people to regulate their own health. The information becomes empowering when someone actually applies the information in his or her life. The classical physician spends a great deal of time educating patients. Once a patient has applied the information and improved her health, the physician serves as a source of further information for emergencies, or as a mentor for reaching even greater levels of health.

The "Fix me" syndrome

Unfortunately, some patients do not want information. They want to be fixed like a car in an auto service center. After spending nearly an hour coaching a patient on diet, exercise changes, and stress reduction, trying to explain why her (mostly junk food) diet was intimately linked with her fatigue, she gave me an exasperated look.

"Can't you just give me some pills?" she asked. "I mean, the last doctor I went to gave me some tablets, and I felt better as long as I was taking them. Can't you just give me something to take?"

Reluctantly, I prescribed some antioxidants, knowing that I was offering a band aid for a much bigger problem. In addition to poor diet and lack of exercise, the patient worked a very stressful job during the day and nursed her terminally ill mother in the evenings. She was overwhelmed at the prospect of making any significant changes in her life. She wanted her health to improve without changing any of the conditions that contributed to her illness.

Perhaps in this situation I needed to start more simply, more slowly in the educative process. And perhaps the patient, at that time in her life, was not ready for a medical model that required her participation. Not every patient is interested in long term health or empowerment. For these patients, drugs and surgery are valid choices.

Drugs versus lifestyle changes

Many people continue to operate in a paradigm engendered by the conventional medical system: "I'm hurting. Give me a pill to take away the pain so I can continue on with my life." The problem with the paradigm is that sometimes the patient's life is the cause of the pain. Simply taking away the pain with a magic bullet pill will not improve health. Even many classical physicians are swayed by the Siren song of symptomatic pain relief. Some prescribe for quick, symptomatic relief and hope the patient will return to address the underlying condition. Others are satisfied with simple pain relief.

Diagnosis and detective work

What this means for you:

Make a list of questions to ask your physician during your next office visit. Bring copies of research you find about your condition or treatment so you can discuss the information together.

Earlier we mentioned the heavy responsibility placed on physicians to accurately diagnose and treat patients. Granted, the accuracy of diagnosis and efficacy of treatment become more important when the medical arsenal is stocked with potentially lethal weapons. Incorrect application of pharmaceutical drugs or surgery can cause a host of side effects and even death. Still, the burden to diagnose accurately 100 percent of the time rests heavily on contemporary physicians. In the world of classical medicine, the physician's responsibility changes somewhat, as does the patient's. The doctor examines, asks, listens, and then makes the most accurate diagnosis possible. She explains her thinking, outlines the other possible causes, and then offers treatment suggestions. The patient then picks up part of the responsibility, realizing that he or she must participate in the treatment plan. The physician and patient may discuss laboratory tests, reviewing the pros and cons of the procedure and weighing the importance of the information against the invasiveness or discomfort of the test. Ideally they make a contract, outlining the treatment and scheduling follow-up visits to evaluate progress.

The re-evaluation periods are particularly important. During these sessions the doctor and patient review progress and adjust the treatment plan as needed. Perhaps the treatment needs to be more aggressive, or the patient may not have been able to implement all of the changes. Some patients halfheartedly follow the plan, or swallow the prescribed pills and forget the rest of the recommendations, then fail to keep the follow-up appointment. "Oh, Dr. So-and-so's treatment didn't work for me. I'm going to see someone else." Or the patient may follow the plan meticulously but make meager progress. The follow-up visit provides both doctor and patient the opportunity to evaluate the effectiveness of the treatment plan and discuss further options.

Usually a classical physician has plan B, C, and D prepared in his or her mind, knowing that each individual is unique, and the first plan may need to be fine-tuned or changed completely. Patients do not understand that a classical physician may have multiple ways of treating one particular condition. Psoriasis, for example, may respond to an herbal formula, a homeopathic remedy, dietary changes, and/or avoidance of inhalant allergies. Most patients are used to the physician who has one plan, one drug, or one procedure to treat a particular ailment. Assuming that the physician has only one

What this means for you:

Keep notes on your response to treatment – you may not remember everything. Usually we are better at noticing when symptoms develop than when they resolve.

approach to offer, the patient moves on to another health care provider and begins the investigative process all over again.

Medicine as a team effort

Patients are often surprised by how long an appointment lasts with a classical medical practitioner. Accustomed to spending only five minutes in the room with a physician, a thirty or sixty minute visit may seem an unaccustomed luxury. Often much of that time is spent gathering information, educating, and answering questions. The doctor may explain a physiological function in the body or outline the progression of a disease. He may give instructions about a particular treatment or review the function of a nutrient in the body. Ideally, if he has done his job well, you will leave with a greater understanding of your body. You now have new understandings and new tools to apply in your life.

In my practice I offer lectures and experiential classes to provide information on topics vital to creating and maintaining health. Once patients have this basic foundation, we can fine tune the information for their particular needs during private visits. The classes save me from repeating the basic information over and over again with each patient individually; instead, we can have more in-depth discussions during

What this means for you:

If the treatment plan you developed with your doctor does not work, contact your physician and ask if he/she has other ideas for treatment before making an appointment with another health care provider.

private consultations.

As the physician's role shifts to educator rather than adjudicator, the relationship with a patient transforms to one of shared exploration and responsibility. The doctor teaches; the patient participates in the application of that knowledge. Together they work as a team with the common goal of health and vibrant aliveness.

> **SECRET #11:**
> **Notice how your life affects your health.**

Almost always several factors contribute to the development of an illness, and usually the most appropriate treatment will be multi-faceted as well. During office visits I ask, "What is going on in your life? Why do think you are ill right now?" Some are surprised. They are not accustomed to having a physician include anything but physical symptoms in their diagnostic work up. Many already know the cause of their illness. Others need coaching and cajoling to understand that their physical bodies are intimately linked with their mental, emotional, and spiritual lives.

I do not mean to imply that all illnesses have an emotional, mental, or spiritual cause. At one time, I was convinced that all illness was due to an issue or issues that a patient was manifesting through a physical illness. Identifying and changing emotional or mental patterns would resolve the physical illness. Over time my thinking has changed. Sometimes people do create diseases to work through "issues." Sometimes people have an iron deficiency because they have an iron deficiency, not because they have some great cosmic lesson to learn. Letting go of the need to find a "metaphysical" cause for every illness has allowed me to be much less judgmental of people. Abandoning my certainty about the causes of disease provides much more room for the great mystery of health and disease to express itself.

Healing occurs on many levels.

The healing process often causes unresolved wounds from the past to resurface. The "wounding" may have occurred on the physical, mental, emotional, or spiritual level. Focusing on healing any aspect can restimulate past hurts as well. The body has enough energy to "clean house," to bring forth, examine, and discharge past garbage. Clearing emotional pain, for example, may be accompanied by the return of a skin rash that plagued the patient during childhood. Healing the rash may be followed by the realization of an unworkable relationship pattern that she is ready to change. The path by which someone returns to wholeness is unique to each individual, although certain patterns of healing may typify that path. While your own journey may differ from this template, you may find shadings of the pattern in your own healing process. This template of healing outlined

---

What this means for you:

When you are ill, consider what else is happening in your life. Do you need to change anything? Do you simply need a rest? Instead of berating yourself, simply notice what is happening.

---

below is common to both Naturopathic and Homeopathic medicines:

The Laws of Cure

Healing occurs
- from inside to outside (internal organs first and skin last)
- from top to bottom (from the head region down to the feet)
- from most recent to most distant (recent symptoms recur first, followed by older symptoms later; in other words, reverse chronological order)

Individualized treatment

Classical medicine diverges from our conventional medical system in its focus on the patient first, rather than the disease. The practitioner sees a human being suffering with a disease, not a disease inhabiting a human body. Conventional medicine's myopic fascination with the disease process has led to major imbalances in the way physicians treat illnesses. The "scientific" method assumes that each person will manifest a particular disease in the same way – every case of a cold is the same, every presentation of ulcerative colitis is the same, every case of sinusitis is the same, and so on, and therefore the treatment should be the same. Research attempts to standardize the treatment according to the illness, not according to the human being; hence, a three hundred pound man with high blood pressure receives the same dose of medicine as a 98-pound woman with high blood pressure. Despite their differences in size, the dosage remains the same. No wonder women tend to have more iatrogenic [ee-at-row-GEN-ic] (physician induced) ill-nesses! They are much more likely to suffer from drug over-doses because researchers conduct the majority of drug testing on white, college aged males, who as a group tend to be physically larger than most women, particularly elderly women.

For patients accustomed to this one-size-fits-all approach to treatment, a classical physician's questions may seem ludicrous. "What kinds of symptoms are you having with the cold?" asks the doctor.

"Well, it's a cold," replies the indignant patient.

"I understand," says the doctor, "and I'm wondering what kinds of symptoms you are having. Are you coughing?"

"Oh, no, not coughing," says the patient, emphatically shaking his head.

"Any nasal congestion?"

"Lots. And today it looks a bit green. Does that mean I have a bacterial infection?"

"Perhaps," says the doctor. "And does the congestion seem to be worse any particular time during the day?"

As the interview continues, the classical physician gathers information about this particular patient's experience of a cold. The hydrotherapy treatments or herbs or homeopathic remedy the physician chooses will be unique to each patient's set of symptoms.

The physician understands that she may see ten patients with a "cold," each with a very different presentation of symptoms, and therefore requiring different treatments.

Research and Classical medicine

Many researchers struggle with how to design studies to test classical medical approaches such as homeopathy or herbs. Recent double-blind, placebo controlled studies have demonstrated the efficacy of homeopathic remedies in treating certain diseases. Despite positive test results, all double-blind studies of homeopathic and other classical treatments share a common weakness: the same remedy is given to different subjects suffering with the same disease. In contrast to this procedure, the homeopathic method of prescribing involves assessing the complete picture and choosing a remedy that best suits that individual. One person with a cough, for example, may also have a sore throat that hurts as if she had a fish bone lodged in the back of the throat and an intense aversion to cold. Another person may have a loose cough in the morning and a dry cough in the evening, feel stifled in a warm room, and better outside in the cool, fresh air. For the first person the classical practitioner might prescribe the homeopathic remedy *Hepar sulph* and for the second *Pulsatilla*.

What this means for you:

Each person develops an illness in their own unique way. Ideally treatment would be individualized to address his or her particular needs.

Whole person, whole planet

Patients treated with natural remedies have a very different impact on the larger environment than those dependent on petroleum-based pharmaceutical drugs. Those who rely on more naturally based treatments understand the importance of caring for the environment. Hydrotherapy treatments rely on clean, pure water for maximum healing effect. Farmers grow optimally nutritious produce in soil replete with humus and the full range of nutrients. Those who rely on herbs for medicine understand that destroying forest habitats diminishes the supply of goldenseal and ginseng, two time-honored herbs that have long been studied for their medicinal properties.

Many herbalists and classical physicians recognize the impact of foraging and "wild crafting" on the native plant populations. Richard Liebmann, N.D., founder of United Plant Savers, is a naturopathic physician dedicated to protecting, replanting, and responsibly harvesting native plant species (see Appendix B for contact information). During this century certain plants have been harvested so heavily that they are now in short supply. Goldenseal, for example, is increasingly difficult to find in the wild. Sharol Tilgner, N.D., owner of Wise Woman Herbals™, recommends substituting the herb *Coptis* (goldthread) or *Mahonia aquafolium* (Oregon graperoot) which have some similar botanical properties. Ironically herbal enthusiasts over-harvested *Coptis* in the late nineteenth century, and responsible herbalists recommended using goldenseal in its stead. Now, a century later, we have gathered too much of the goldenseal and are shifting back to *Coptis* for its bitter and anti-microbial properties.

"If people want to address what's happening to the Earth," says Dr. Tilgner, "they really need to look at the over-population issue. Even though there are things that can be substituted, kind of, for goldenseal – you never can find all of the qualities of a particular plant in another – you've just transferred the problem from goldenseal to *Coptis*. We're looking at the symptoms – goldenseal disappearing or global warming – but not at the real root of the problem. There are a lot of us here. The real solution is to reduce our population."

Earth remedies versus synthetic drugs

In contrast to the environmentally dependent natural remedies, most pharmaceutical companies derive drugs from a petroleum source. When countries go to war over oil reserves, their reasons for fighting include not only energy resources but also the base for synthesizing many prescription medicines. Most drug companies are more interested in the synthetic molecules they can derive from petroleum products than they are in promoting naturally occurring products.

Money in part explains the fascination with synthetically derived drugs. Until the mid-1980s,

What this means for you:

Even "natural" remedies impact the Earth's health. Use only what you need. Support groups that responsibly harvest and replant native herbs. Consider growing your own medicinal herbs.

no one could patent naturally occurring substances in the body; hence, a synthetically derived molecule that mimics but does not duplicate something the body makes is more attractive to the pharmaceutical industry than making an exact duplicate of a substance in the body. A synthetic progestin, for example, mimics but does not duplicate the body's progesterone. Because the molecule is altered, the message that the drug transmits is altered, producing a wide range of side effects. Pharmaceutical companies do know how to make an exact duplicate of progesterone, one that is "bio-identical" (exactly the same as the molecule the body produces), but they cannot patent the bio-identical progesterone. Instead, they patent and manufacture synthetic progestins, thereby increasing their profits.

Currently pharmaceutical companies are also not allowed to patent naturally occurring plant substances. Without a patent to guarantee profitability, the companies are reluctant to invest funds in studies that would prove the benefits of plant medicines. Unlike scientists in the United States, German researchers have invested time and money in studying the medicinal benefits of plants and have produced many excellent scientific studies on plant functions and properties.

Naturally derived remedies strengthen our connection with the Earth. Those who rely on petroleum-based pharmaceutical medicines unwittingly support a system of greed and global manipulation to ensure their production. An astute classical physician understands that the vitality of her medicines is allied with the health of the environment. Treating the whole person may include remedying the environment as well. Whole people live in a vital, thriving ecosystem.

SECRET #12:
Make daily investments in your health.

What this means for you:

Everything you do to support the health of the environment in turn supports your own health. Healthy people live in a healthy environment.

Preventive care requires studying health as closely as the processes of disease. Occasionally researchers set out to discover the principles of health, focusing on cultures with virile, long-lived elders. Most of the studies dwell on the physical environment, food, or water supply of the centenarians. Their research has uncovered fascinating clues pointing to elements that promote longevity, such as subtle differences in local water supply (Flannagan), mineral content of the soil and plants (Wallach), and nutrient-rich local foods. Few also include the influence of the unseen and immeasurable, such as emotional support, cultural attitudes, and spiritual understanding, yet their overall quest is laudable – uncovering the roots of health by examining the healthiest and longest lived of the species.

Conventional medicine aims for survival; classical medicine aims for optimal health. Our government's current "preventive" medicine program encourages immunization for young children. To a certain extent, not withstanding the potentially devastating impact of certain immunizations on later health, vaccination is a worthy goal. As the sum total of a preventive treatment program, however, immunizing young children is a feeble gesture. True preventive medicine requires making daily investments in our health – eating foods that nourish our bodies, exercising, developing loving relationships and supportive communities, and contributing to the health of the Earth.

A country focused on preventive medicine would create a culture that viewed health as "sexy" and as desirable as a fast, shiny car or an expensive home. Such a society would invest in services and products that increased their own health while minimizing environmental impact. Celebrations would include delicious, well cooked organic foods rather than sugar-hydrogenated-fats-and-preservatives-surprise! junk foods. People would celebrate in ways that enhanced rather than destroyed their health. Equating celebration with life-destroying activities negates the purpose of festivities – to affirm and celebrate accomplishments, and to honor a person or action.

Healthy people live in healthy environments. Because human health is inseparable from the health of the planet, preventative medicine means working for clean air, land, and water. Our human health is inseparable from the health of the planet.

Lace up your boots and get ready to go

This book is a journey, an odyssey intended to support you in the creation of lifelong health. Initially we will focus on your vision of health. What does health look like for you? Do you want to be healthy for a lifetime? You will have a chance to evaluate your health, developing a clear, concise picture of your current situation. Next we will explore the foundations of health, increasing your knowledge base so that you can make effective choices to create health. Finally, we will review your health goals and evaluate your actions to make sure they support your desired vision of health.

For best results, find a physician who can be your ally in customizing the information for your particular needs. Collaborate with a health care provider who will work with you in applying the information in this book to achieve your health goals. For additional support, see the contact information in Appendix B.

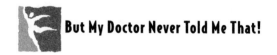

NOTES:

CHAPTER 3

The Oracle of Hygieia: Divining the Secrets of Lifelong Health

Hygieia, Greek goddess of health, blessed her followers with vibrant health. Hygieia's devotees, however, did more than simply pay homage to the goddess. Her followers took inspiration from Hygieia and followed her example to create lifelong health.

Have you secretly harbored a vision of yourself in vibrant health? Have you hidden those images because you were unsure of how to realize them? Many health care providers tell us that we're "just getting older." The changes in our bodies are inevitable, so why bother trying to challenge the status quo?

Are you uncomfortable with this fatalistic view of health? Do you want fully vibrant health, no matter what your age? Many people want healthy bodies, healthy minds, and healthy lives, not just the absence of disease. The truth is they want health, no matter what the current condition of their bodies.

"Be realistic," hisses the Voice of Caution. "I'm not 25 anymore. Do you really think I'm going to eat bean sprouts for breakfast and lose that whale blubber around my waist?"

SECRET #1:
Choose to be healthy.

What this
means for
you:

Know where you

want to go in life.

What do you want

to create?

"When you go to the bus station," explains Phyllis Rodin, an 84-year-old friend, "you've got to know where you're going before you can buy a ticket. You can't just say to the person at the counter, 'I want a ticket.' You have to know where you are going. The same thing is true in your life – you've got to know where you're going before you can buy a ticket. That's the ticket!"

One of the first secrets in journeying toward health is choosing to be healthy. Have you chosen to be healthy?

Motivation

As you consider whether or not you want to be healthy, ask yourself, "Why do I want to be healthy?" Most people have never asked themselves this question. "Well, of course I'm supposed to want to be healthy," you may say to yourself. "Doesn't everyone want to be healthy?"

SECRET #2:
Being healthy serves your life visions.

For most people, health is a necessary prerequisite to create what truly matters to them. Without health, they cannot bring those visions to fruition.

Consider what is most important to you in your life. What matters to you? What do you want to create? For the moment set aside thoughts about whether or not those creations are possible; instead, tell yourself the truth about what you really want in life.

Although many people desire health, each person has his or her own reason for wanting to be healthy. For Ann, choosing health may be a way of pleasing her spouse. George may choose health to avoid heart disease or cancer. Sarah Jane may desire health so that she can create what matters most to her. Paul may choose health to support his life vision of raising a family and pursuing a painting career.

Your motivation for choosing health impacts your ability to create health. Choosing health to serve your life vision fundamentally differs from avoiding illness, problem solving, or pleasing others.

Pitfalls on the journey to creating health: avoiding, problem solving, and placating

---

SECRET #3:
Strategies to avoid illness do not lead
to lifelong health.

Consider again the original question: have you made a choice to be healthy? Many people pursue all kinds of "health programs," dietary approaches, and exercise routines, yet they have never chosen to be healthy. These people may choose to participate in programs to avoid certain illnesses or avoid losing their health. When they avoid something, however, what do they end up with? An absence of something. Remember that full, vibrant health is more than the absence of disease, more than the avoidance of future illness.

Problem solving versus creating

Creating something is radically different from problem solving. When you solve a problem, the difficulty "goes away." Instead of creating something new, you have eliminated something you do not want.

Most medical systems focus on eliminating problems – slay the symptom. Avoid illness. Prevent disease. All of these approaches are problem-solving strategies. None of these methods focus on what you want to create; instead, they address what you want to avoid or eliminate. As you create health, you may very well employ medical services to fulfill your vision of health. The framework in which you apply those treatments, however, varies completely from the problem-solving approach.

Avoiding the ravages of disease

My friend Mary called shortly after her annual gynecological exam with the news that her physician had found a breast lump. She wanted me to verify her physician's explanation of the mammogram report.

"Here are the test results," she said, reading them

over the phone. "Is my doctor telling me the truth, or is he trying to make me feel better so I don't worry?" Filled with medical jargon, the mammogram report basically stated that she probably had an aggressive, malignant tumor. The physician could not make a definitive diagnosis until after he had completed a biopsy of the tumor.

During the following month Mary's life changed radically. Her tumor was malignant, and she had reams of decisions to make. In addition to having surgery to remove the breast lump, Mary changed her diet and began a natural supplement regimen. She decided to pursue chemotherapy treatments but refused radiation because of its poor track record in treating her particular type of cancer.

One Saturday afternoon Mary called in a panic, wanting to know if she could take more of the acidophilus supplement her doctor had recommended. She was struggling with candida overgrowth in her vagina and on her skin that caused tremendous itching. Chemotherapy wipes out all the flora in the digestive tract, providing the perfect environment for certain bacteria and fungi to flourish. I tried to refer her back to her own doctor, but she was insistent.

I explained that the doctor probably had recommended taking only a small amount of acidophilus rather than following the full program because she would wipe out the flora all over again with the next round of chemotherapy.

"Will taking more acidophilus hurt me?" asked Mary.

"No," I explained, "but you're wasting your money. Your doctor suggested you take a small amount because the next round of chemotherapy will destroy the microorganisms you are replacing now."

"I understand I'm probably wasting my money taking more of the acidophilus," said Mary. "What can I do now?"

I empathized with Mary. "Chemotherapy is amazing stuff. It shuts down everything in the body. That's its nature. Chemotherapy stops all cell division, in the tumor and in the rest of the body."

"Well, I didn't really have any choice," she said, sighing.

"It's your body, isn't it?" I asked.

"Yes," she said. "But my family was totally freaked out when I told them I was thinking about not doing chemotherapy. They just wouldn't listen to me. I had to do this."

"Does your body belong to you or your family?" I asked again.

"It's more complicated than that," she replied.

What this means for you:

Avoiding illness will not create health.

Mary is right. We often face extremely complicated health care decisions, particularly if we are struggling with a chronic disease. Mary hoped to elude the cancer and avoid her family's distress about her health care choices. Usually we are busy trying to avoid undesirable circumstances. Rather than moving toward a vision of health, we are running desperately from a feared condition.

"Solving the problem" of breast cancer (or any other condition) will not necessarily create health. Someone with breast cancer, however, could choose to create health. The fact that she has breast cancer becomes part of the evaluation of her current health status. Breast cancer becomes a feature in the landscape rather than the sole focus of her attention.

Some women with breast cancer can create their vision of health, while others cannot. Women with breast cancer or anyone else with a serious illness will have a greater chance of creating health if they desire health in order to fulfill other important life goals. Rather than solving the problem of cancer, their health care choices support the creation of what truly matters to them.

> What this means for you:
>
> *You can choose to create health even if you have a chronic disease or terminal illness.*

Resolving a problem will not create health

Ellen, another woman diagnosed with breast cancer, spent her last months desperately trying to gain her father's recognition. Ellen had spent most of her life trying to win her father's approval, and her illness only intensified the quest. Rather than focusing on what she wanted to create, Ellen dedicated herself to manipulating her father, trying to force him to recognize her and thereby validate her life. Ellen immersed herself in problem solving. She was certain she could fix all of her problems by winning her father's recognition. Ellen's "solution" depended on something outside herself that ultimately she could not control – her father's opinion of her.

Of course many factors influence someone's recovery from cancer or any other major illness. I could not say definitively that Ellen's problem-solving orientation was the sole reason for the rapid progression of her disease. Someone struggling with a terminal illness, however, has a greater chance of recovery if she chooses health in order to serve her life visions. The process of creating is essentially a life-affirming pursuit. Creating engages our life force, our innate regenerative capacity, as we birth new projects, objects, or states of being into the world. This creative focus seems to revive the body's generative abilities as well. We can co-create health in tandem with the realization of our passions and life visions. Choosing health does not guarantee recovery, but choosing health in order to create what matters most can improve the chances of survival.

What do you really want?

Someone with a terminal illness may argue he can never have vibrant health, so why should he bother choosing it? Part of the choosing process is to tell yourself the truth about what you really want. Even if he never achieves full health, at least the chronically ill person does not have the additional burden of lying to himself about what matters most to him. He can tell himself the truth about what he wants and choose health regardless of whether or not he can realize his vision.

What this means for you:

Creating health is fundamentally different from solving health problems.

Creating brings something into being that never existed before; problem solving eliminates an unwanted condition or circumstance.

Simply choosing health does not guarantee you will achieve health. You will not know until you take action whether or not you can achieve optimal health. Choosing health, however, increases your ability to take appropriate action, evaluate your progress, and adjust your actions as necessary.

Oscillating structures - the "yo-yo" syndrome

Health strategies designed to minimize risks or circumvent disease soon lose momentum. Any improvement in health diminishes the reason to continue the program: "Hey, my blood pressure is down!" says Bill. "The doctor says I've lowered my risk for heart disease. I'm more relaxed, not so scared anymore – why should I keep up this walking program?"

If avoidance is the motivation for taking action, the greater the distance from the feared event, the less reason you have to take action. In the avoidance strategy, the closer you are to the feared event (e.g. illness, stroke, death), the more action you will take. As soon as health improves, however, the impetus to take action diminishes.

After lapsing into his old ways, Bill's blood pressure probably will rise again. The pounds he struggled so hard to lose will return . . . plus a few more. As Bill's health deteriorates, the desire to improve his health increases. He "motivates" himself and returns to his healthy diet and exercise program.

> What this means for you:
>
> *Telling yourself the truth about what you want, regardless of whether or not you think you can have it, takes less energy than trying to talk yourself out of your deepest desires.*

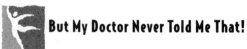

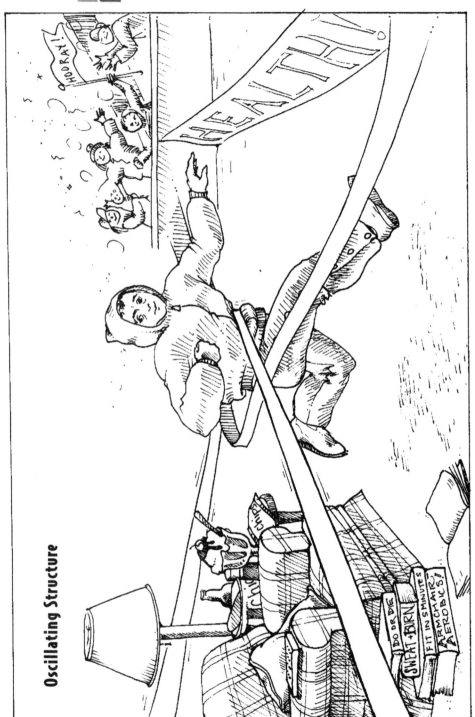

Oscillating Structure

This familiar pattern of see-sawing toward and away from your desired goals is what Robert Fritz, author of *The Path of Least Resistance*, calls an "oscillating structure." Bill truly wants good health. He also really wants to eat rich food and avoid exercise. These two goals are in conflict. Bill can't have both health and an overly rich diet and no exercise. Imagine this man standing between his two opposite desires – health on one side and his familiar foods and lack of exercise on the other. Imagine a rubber band connecting him to health, and another rubber band connecting him to his beloved foods and his easy chair. The conflict generates a pendulum-like series of actions for the would-be health enthusiast. As soon as he moves toward "health," the pull toward the opposite desire becomes stronger. He overcomes the opposite pull by "motivating" himself, pumping himself up with books, audiocassettes, and declarations to all of his friends about his goals. The closer he moves to health, however, the stronger the pull toward his beloved foods and comfortable chair. When he follows the stronger pull, abandoning his exercise program and resuming his usual diet, the pull toward health will be stronger. He resolves to "try harder," buys several new books and a video for motivation, and begins yet another swing in the direction of health. He will choose one goal or the other, depending on where he is in the oscillating structure.

What this means for you:

In an oscillating structure, you may near or even achieve your health goals, but eventually you will return to your former habits and state of health.

Many program participants are mystified when they return to their former habits, regain weight, stop exercising, and feel fatigued. No amount of motivation, inspiration, or perspiration will propel you toward your vision of health if you are focused on preventing disease. Choosing health is a vital step toward the creation of health, yet any attempt to "fix" an oscillating structure by choosing health only reinforces the oscillation. Unfortunately we can not problem-solve our way out of an oscillating structure. For someone swinging back and forth, choosing health may be yet another attempt at fixing, resolving, or altering the oscillating structure. Within a resolving structure (see page 94), however, the choice to create health catalyzes the fulfillment of your vision.

The "do or die" syndrome

Many people in an oscillating structure will abandon their health goals at the first "transgression." "Darn," says the man in the oscillating structure, devouring hot fudge and ice cream. "I thought I was going to make it this time. I told myself this was it, do or die. I was going to lower my blood pressure or else! Well, I've blown it now. All that good work, and now I'm eating this hot fudge sundae. Sigh. I might as well order a steak and some fries and a milkshake. What the hell – I've blown it already, right? I think I'll make reservations for Bob's Super Pig-Out Buffet tomorrow night. I mean, I haven't eaten there for at least a month!"

Resolving structures – moving toward your goals

Someone who has chosen to be healthy may take the very same actions as a health enthusiast operating in the avoidance strategy. The person who has chosen health, however, is moving toward a desired outcome rather than away from what she fears. When health improves, she will continue walking, even though her cholesterol levels have dropped. She will continue eating healthy food, even though her cholesterol levels have returned to normal. "I feel great!" she proclaims. "I want to feel this way when I'm 75, so I'm keeping up my walking program and eating healthy food. I haven't felt this good since I was 16!"

Robert Fritz describes this movement as a "resolving structure." Here the person is not oscillating between two opposite goals. Instead, she has chosen her vision of health and is making choices to support the realization of that vision. Sure, she may still love hot fudge sundaes and sitting for hours in front of the TV watching her favorite sit-coms. Her choice for health, however, creates a hierarchy for her decisions. She may want to eat the hot fudge sundae, but she chooses an apple instead. She doesn't pretend she doesn't love ice cream, but rather makes a choice for what she wants. "Ooooh," she says to herself. "That hot fudge sundae looks so good. I love the way the hot fudge softens the top of the ice cream, and the chopped nuts on top, and the way the whipped cream melts in my mouth . . . yeah, and here's the apple in the fridge. Yep, I'm choosing the apple. I've decided to keep my cholesterol down, so it's apples for me."

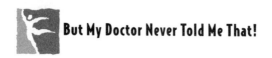

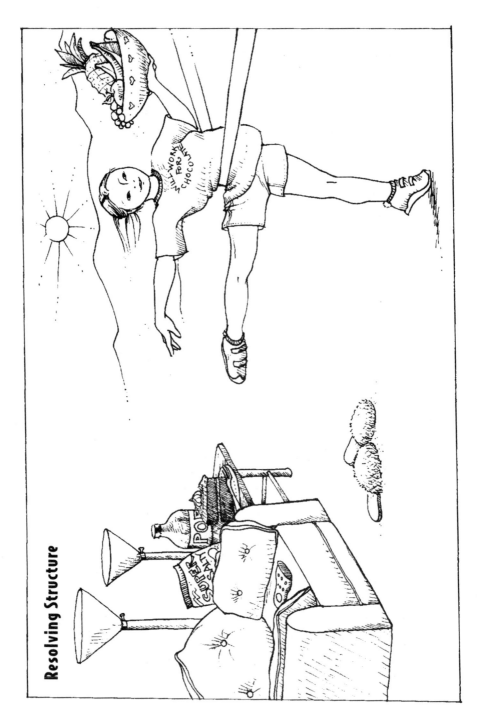

Resolving Structure

If this woman does choose at some point to eat a hot fudge sundae, a pile of fried chicken, gravy, and biscuits smothered with butter, she most likely will resume her healthy eating habits. The grease binge is a temporary deviation, not a complete oscillation in her journey toward health. She stuffs himself at the family reunion and spends the day lolling around in the shade, visiting with family. The next day, however, she resumes her exercise program and healthy diet. She still desires health and continues making choices for her health, despite the temporary detour. Her choice is for a lifetime, not just a short term goal (e.g. lowering her cholesterol levels).

> **SECRET #4:**
> **Create a clear picture of health.**

What does health look like to you? Do you have an image of yourself in full, vibrant health? Take a few minutes to compose a clear picture for yourself (either mentally or on paper). Sketch in as much detail as possible. Paint the picture as completely and boldly as you can. For right now, forget about whether or not your picture is "realistic." Many of the great innovations of our time never would have been completed if their creators had insisted on being "realistic." Just tell yourself the truth about how you want to look, how you want to feel, and what a healthy life looks like for you. Include all the elements of health that are important to you, e.g. physical, mental, emotional, spiritual, and environmental health.

As you create this picture, ask yourself the following questions:

1. "Have I told myself the truth about what I really want?" For the moment, forget about what you think is possible. Just tell yourself the unedited truth about what you want. You may want to lose every ounce of cellulite on your thighs and buttocks but hesitate to include that detail in the vision for a variety of reasons, e.g. "Sigh . . . I've had jiggling, chubby thighs since I was four years old – that will never change." The fact that you've always had chubby thighs does not change your desire to have firm thighs. Be honest with yourself about what you really want.

2. "Have I diminished the vision so that I'm more comfortable with it?" Diminishing your goals may make you feel more comfortable in the short term ("Phew, I'm not as far away as I thought!"), but in the long run you lose the full power of your original vision.

3. "Do I have specific goals that I would recognize if I reached them?" Create a vision that you can accurately measure. Each aspect of the vision will have its own standard of measurement. "Weigh 130 pounds," for example, is a very different vision from "Have 19 percent body fat." The first vision requires a scale. The second calls for a body composition machine OR underwater test to determine the percentage of body fat. You will know if you have a

vague goal if you cannot find a good standard of measurement. "Lose some weight" or "Bring down my blood pressure" are not specific goals. How much is "some" weight? Two pounds? Two hundred pounds? Does "bringing down" blood pressure mean diastolic or systolic blood pressure (the upper and lower numbers)? Both? How much do you want to reduce blood pressure? "Consistent blood pressure readings of 120/80 mm Hg for a month" is a much more specific vision with a clearly defined measurement.

4. "If I could inhabit this vision, would I take it?" This question reminds you to fill in any details or discard any extraneous elements in your vision. Maybe you discover that your desire for a 26-inch waist was the result of your brother's incessant childhood teasing. Is that what you really want now? If the answer is "Yes!" by all means include it in the vision. If not, discard that detail. Maybe life just isn't worth living unless you have a garden or live near the ocean – make sure you include all of the elements of health that are important to you.

5. "Do I choose to be healthy?" Remember the power of choosing health.

SECRET #5:
Know where you are in relationship to
your vision.

As with any journey, you need a good idea of where you are before you begin. Imagine wanting to drive from

Los Angeles to New York City but telling yourself you are in Seattle, Washington. If you start making decisions as if you were in Seattle, you have very little chance of reaching New York.

Where are you now? What is your state of health? Answer that question as accurately and completely as possible. You may choose to have an annual physical to measure the basics, e.g. blood pressure, reflexes, blood work, and a Pap smear for women. In addition, gather information about your current lifestyle – what are you eating, how much are you exercising, how much stress do you have in your life, and how effectively are you coping? Use the questionnaires and charts on pages 100-105 to help you create an accurate picture of where you are now in relation to your health goals.

As you make lifestyle changes, the current health picture will change. You will need to reassess your state of health as you progress. Having an accurate picture of your current state helps you to choose appropriate next steps.

For the next week, keep track of your diet and exercise. You will find additional copies of the diet diary and exercise journal at the end of the book. You are welcome to photocopy these charts so that you can use them again and again to get an accurate "bead" on your current state of health.

In addition to reviewing your diet and exercise habits, I also highly recommend getting a copy of *The Stress Map*. This invaluable tool allows you to assess four aspects of stress in your life: your environment (work and personal), coping responses, inner world (thoughts and feelings), and signals of distress. The last section offers suggestions to address specific areas of "strain" or "burn out." Photocopy the "map" in the center so that you can re-use it in the future. You can order *The Stress Map* at your local bookstore or directly from Newmarket Press: 18 East 48th St., New York, NY 10017. (212) 832-3575.

**SECRET #6:
Work with structural tension.**

The disparity between your current state and the place you want to be generates a tension that moves you toward your destination. Robert Fritz in his book *The Path of Least Resistance* calls this "structural tension." Think of the anticipation at the beginning of a road trip. You have packed the car, studied the road map, and chosen your route. Finally you turn on the ignition and roll down the driveway. You imagine the skyscrapers of New York and that final drive across one of the bridges onto the island of Manhattan. For the moment, you are aware of the hot, hazy skies and palm-lined boulevards of Los Angeles.

The difference between your current location and your final destination creates a tension. Imagine a huge rubber band stretching across the continent, connecting your car in Los Angeles with your desired destination in New York. On a road trip, you may experience this tension as "anticipation." A painter may recognize this tension as a sense of urgency or increased focus on

DIET JOURNAL for _____ **Beginning Date** _____

The purpose of this diary is to provide you and your doctor with an unbiased record of your normal eating habits. Simply eat your typical diet and record what you eat for seven days in sucession. Under breakfast, lunch, and dinner columns list food and drink ingredients and amounts. Under BM, list bowel movement times. Under Notes, list symptoms such as mood swings, indigestion, headaches, fatigue, etc. Remember to include snacks.

Include supplements (brand name, ingredients, potency):

Breakfast DAY 1	Lunch	Dinner	BM Times	Notes
DAY 2				
DAY 3				

	Breakfast	Lunch	Dinner	BM Times	Notes
DAY 4					
DAY 5					
DAY 6					
DAY 7					

Additional Notes _____

Exercise Adherence Questionnaire

Directions: Check each statement that applies to you.

Beliefs

____I am too old to exercise.

____Exercise only helps if you do a lot, and I'm not an iron man!

____I think I am uncoordinated and feel too embarrassed to exercise.

____Exercise is all work and no play.

____I will be injured if I begin to exercise.

____Sweating is disgusting.

____Exercise is good for my health.

My Style

____I drive myself hard.

____If something seems too hard, I will give up.

When I relapse from my exercise program due to injury or illness:

____I probably won't start again.

____I will ridicule myself for stopping my exercise program.

____I will certainly begin exercising again.

____I prefer to exercise alone.

____I love team sports.

____I would exercise more consistently if I worked out with a group
or a friend.

____I want immediate results or I will not stick to my program.

Exercise Adherence Questionnaire

My Support Team

___ The people I live with think exercise is silly.

___ Even though no one at home supports my exercise program, I have a friend or family member who will.

___ The people I live with will be neutral about my exercise program.

___ The people I live with will be encouraging of my exercise program.

___ I care what other people think of me.

___ I don't give a hoot about what others think.

My choices

___ I have chosen to exercise to support my vision of health.

___ I can't exercise now . . . . maybe later.

___ Not now, not ever!

My History

___ I was usually the last one picked for school teams.

___ I have been made fun of playing sports or wearing a bathing suit.

___ I was a super jock in high school or college.

___ Moderate exercise has always been part of my daily life.

EXERCISE JOURNAL for _____   **Beginning Date** _____

The purpose of this diary is to provide you and your doctor with an unbiased record of your normal exercise habits. Simply follow your typical exercise routine and record what you do for seven days in sucession. For every day list the amount and type of exercise you do using the following descriptions. **Aerobic exercise (AE):** rhythmic, continuous exercise using the large muscles of the body (legs) that deepens breathing and increases the heart beat to target heart rate. Examples: walking, jogging, running, swimming, rowing. **Strength-building exercise (SBE):** resistance exercise that increases muscle strength. Examples: isometrics, calisthenics, weight lifting, sprinting. **Stretching exercise (SE):** stretching and holding muscles at just less than the point of discomfort. Examples: yoga. **Activities of Daily Living (ADL):** activities at work or at home that require movement, e.g. typing, vacuuming, gardening, driving, doing laundry.

		Responses to exercise. (Muscle strains after certain kinds of exercise, enjoyment or dislike of particular types of exercise, etc.)
DAY 1 (AE) – (SBE) – (SE) – (ADL) –		
DAY 2		
DAY 3		

Responses to exercise. (Muscle strains after certain kinds of exercise, enjoyment or dislike of particular types of exercise etc.)	
DAY 4 (AE) – (SBE) – (SE) – (ADL) –	
DAY 5	
DAY 6	
DAY 7	

Additional Notes _____ _____

her work. All creators recognize this pull between their desired creation and their current situation. As a creator of health, you may recognize this "tension" as a powerful force that propels you toward your desired vision of health. You can maintain this structural tension by accurately observing your current state while simultaneously holding an image of your desired state of health.

Vision develops organically

Some people have a hard time envisioning what they have never experienced. If you have never known vibrant health, how can you envision yourself as healthy? Developing a vision for health may be an ongoing process. Consider the development of a baby in the womb. Imagine being pregnant but not knowing exactly what the baby will look like. You may not even know if the baby is a girl or a boy. As the baby develops, you can feel movement inside. Eventually you can trace the outlines of the baby's limbs poking against your belly; you begin to know its shape. Not until the baby is born, however, will you know all of the details of this newly emerging being.

The creation process inherently involves mystery. We can't know every step of the process in advance. The seed of vision grows within us. We nourish that seed with deliberate choices, "fortuitous" meetings, and unexpected intuitions.

Imagine choosing to grow peas in your spring garden. As you press the seeds into the earth and tamp down the sodden spring soil, you cannot foresee the outcome. Only in time do you witness the growth and finally the fruition of that seed. The action steps you take along the way, such as watering, weeding, and mulching, effect the final outcome of the spring planting. As every gardener regretfully knows, however, planting a seed does not guarantee its survival. The action steps increase the likelihood of the seed/vision coming to fruition, but they cannot guarantee the outcome.

What this means for you:

Your vision of health probably will grow and change over time.

The Journey to Health

You will be using the following chart throughout the book to assess your current location and your vision of health (desired destination). After much thought, I carefully chose the word "journey" to describe this exploration of health. A "map" or "path" implies an already established course and a known destination. A journey, however, may require forging a completely new route. Your journey to health will be unique to you, shaped by your personal vision of health. Perhaps you will follow established pathways to create your vision of health. Your vision may require you to bushwhack into unknown territory or combine the known and unknown byways. I cannot offer a pre-determined pathway with a guaranteed destination. Your own vision of health has more power, truth, and passion than any ready-made, one-size-fits-all program I could present to you. Instead, I offer tools to assist you in navigating on your own journey to health.

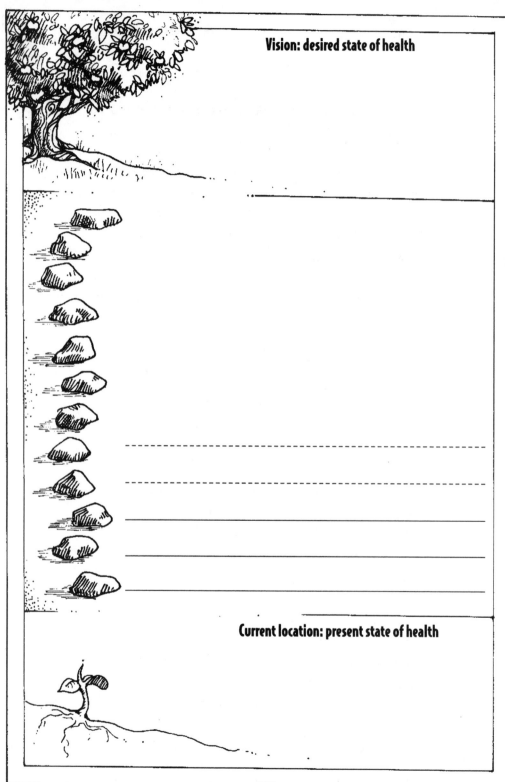

Vision: desired state of health

Current location: present state of health

> **In the following exercise, complete the Journey to Health chart in seven steps:**

1. Describe your destination (the state of health you desire).

2. Accurately describe your current location (your current state of health).

3. Notice the difference between where you are and where you want to be.

4. Simultaneously hold an image of your desired state and your current state of health. Notice the structural tension generated by the disparity between the two pictures.

5. Ask yourself, "If I could have my desired state of health, would I take it?"

6. If the answer is "Yes," then CHOOSE that state of health. "I choose . . ." and describe what you desire.

7. Fill in action steps that will move you toward your destination.

SECRET #7:

Make choices that support your vision of health.

What this means for you:

Create, evaluate, and adjust. You will be modifying your action steps as your progress in the creation of your vision.

As soon as you have a clear destination and a well-defined current location, you often think of steps you can take to fulfill your vision. These "steps" are secondary choices that support your primary choice – to be healthy. Write down as many steps as occur to you. These action steps arise from reviewing your final destination, clarifying your current position, and then defining the discrepancy between the two locations.

Create, evaluate, and adjust

Keep in mind that you will be adjusting these secondary choices over time as you progress on your journey toward health. You may discover, for example, a particular exercise program that better fits your goals than the exercise you have been doing. After beginning the new program, evaluate the effect of your actions. Has the exercise program moved you toward your vision? Has your health improved as a result of the program? How has your health improved? Remember the importance of having accurate measurements to determine the effectiveness of your actions, e.g. blood pressure readings, body composition tests, or energy levels. The action steps are flexible, subject to evaluation and adjustment. New steps will occur to you as you continue on the journey toward health.

Example of completing the Journey to Health chart

56 year old Harry has been reflecting on his life visions. Harry realizes he wants to be healthy in order to do the things he loves most: working in the garden, hiking, and making love with his partner. Harry knows he feels better, has more energy, and moves more easily when his body fat is around 17 percent. He longs to have enough energy to work in the garden four times a week (three nights after he returns home from work and at least part of one day each weekend), go for a hike three times a month, and make love with his partner at least twice a week.

At his last doctor's visit 2 months ago, Harry's blood pressure was 165/95 mm Hg. He periodically checks his own blood pressure and averages about 160/95. His body composition is 23 percent fat. For the last six months Harry has been too tired to even think about making love. He falls into bed exhausted at 9 P.M. but can't fall asleep until 11 P.M. He sleeps fitfully, gets out of bed at 6 A.M.., and jump starts the coffee maker. Armed with a large mug of coffee and a pastry, he leaves the house at 6:30 A.M. and spends an hour on the congested freeway driving to work. He grinds through the day attending meetings, answering phone calls, and doing paper work. At noon he eats a hoagie sandwich and a cola delivered by the local deli. By 3 P.M. he barely can keep his eyes open, despite having drunk eight cups of coffee. At 4:30 P.M. he leaves the office and spends 90 minutes

(example continued on page 113)

Vision: desired state of health

Harry's first rendition of his Journey to Health chart might look like this: I want to be healthy enough to live the life I want. My standards of measurement (SOM): a consistent blood pressure reading of 125/80 mm Hg, 17 percent body fat, work in the garden four times a week (three times during the week and once on the weekend), hike twice a month, and make love with my partner twice a week.

Action steps on the road to health.

Practice with Deep Relaxation tape five times a week. Completed by _____

Eliminate coffee. Completed by _____

Eat beans for breakfast. Completed by _____

Exercise at lunchtime and during breaks for a total of 30 minutes per day. Completed by _____

Take public transportation to work (increases reading time, reduces stress of rush hour commute). Completed by _____

Practice good sleep hygiene. Completed by _____

Eliminate simple carbohydrates. Completed by _____

Eat three servings of whole grains per day. Completed by _____

Eliminate red meat. Completed by _____

Eat fish three times a week. Completed by _____

17 percent body fat. Completed by _____

Schedule "dates" to make love with my partner when we are not tired or stressed. Completed by _____

Current location: present state of health

Currently I cannot live the life I want. Blood pressure: 165/95 mm Hg. Body composition: 23 percent body fat. Sex: 6 months ago. Hiking: two years ago. Sleep: seven hours, not rested on waking. Diet: 8 cups of coffee per day; lots of simple carbohydrates; some meat; and few vegetables, fruits, or complex carbohydrates. Exercise: no aerobic, strength building, or stretching exercise. Energy (10 = high): 3/10.

driving through rush-hour traffic. When he arrives home at 6 P.M., he looks at the overgrown garden, groans, and retreats to the sofa for an hour's nap. He wakes at 7 P.M., greets his partner, and sits down to a big pasta dinner. He watches a couple of TV shows. At 9 P.M., too sleepy to watch the next show, Harry crawls into bed and lies staring at the ceiling until he finally falls asleep around 11 P.M.

Following the Yellow Brick Road – evaluating your action steps

As you create your action steps, ask yourself the following questions:

- Will this action step move me toward my vision of health? What part of my vision?
- Is the action step specific enough? Do I have an accurate way of measuring the results?
- Will I recognize the result when I see it?
- Have I specified a date by which I will complete this step? Having a specific date helps you organize your actions. If Harry decided to reduce body fat to 17 percent in five years, he would take different actions than if he decided to complete that step in 12 months.
- Which action step is most important right now? Choose the most important action steps first.

Someone with diabetes, for example, might focus first on reducing and stabilizing blood sugar levels by eliminating simple sugars, increasing beans in the diet, and supplementing chromium.

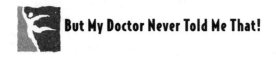

Where am I going next? (Always have a place to go)

The next three chapters will assist you in refining your action steps. The exercises you have completed in this chapter provide both an accurate description of your current state of health and an accurate baseline by which to assess your progress. Embarking on a new journey, you probably have lots of questions: What will I eat? Will the terrain be friendly? Will I have companions along the way? Stay tuned for more secrets to help make your journey a success.

CHAPTER 4

Secrets for Nourishing Your Body

The digestive system literally is the center of the human body. During embryonic development, we begin as tubes that quickly branch and become the major systems of the body. The digestive system consists of a long, elaborate conduit extending from mouth to anus and serves as one of our primary interfaces with the world. Through this passageway we absorb nutrients and discard wastes. In a sense, our bodies are fancy tubes with appendages attached. We can live without arms and legs, but we cannot survive without the digestive system.

SECRET #1:
Know the territory (of the digestive tract).

Let's take a tour of the digestive system, following a bite of a favorite morsel through this miraculously constructed pipe. The first stage of digestion occurs in the mouth, where enzymes in the saliva begin to break down carbohydrates. Chewing also breaks the food into smaller pieces, making the nutrients more available to the rest of the digestive tract. "Chew your drink and drink your food" – in other words, chew food until it becomes liquid, and swish liquid around in the mouth to mix with saliva before swallowing. After we chew food, it passes through the esophagus into the stomach. This movement stimulates peristalsis [pair-is-TAHL-sis], a series of wave-like contractions along the entire digestive tract that ensures the food continues to move through the entire system. The cardiac sphincter [SFINK-ter], a ring-shaped muscle, serves as a gate between the esophagus and stomach.

"Cooking" food

From Chinese medical perspective, the stomach "cooks" food, preparing it for absorption in the rest of the digestive tract. Keep in mind the Chinese describe the body more poetically than western medicine does. In a sense, though, our western understanding of stomach acid breaking down proteins parallels the Chinese view of "cooking" food in the stomach. Recent research suggests that some stomach ulcers result from lack of, rather than excess, acid production. If the stomach does not produce enough hydrochloric acid, certain bacteria may overgrow and colonize the stomach wall. An overgrowth of the bacteria Helicobacter pylori, for example, can cause stomach ulcers and chronic stomach irritation. We need adequate levels of hydrochloric acid production for the stomach to function optimally.

Chief cells, the same cells in the stomach that produce hydrochloric acid, also secrete intrinsic factor (IF), a substance necessary for the absorption of vitamin B12. Vital for normal cell division and healthy nerves, a lack of B12 can cause fatigue, depression, macrocytic anemia, and tingling in the hands and feet. Many older people do not secrete enough hydrochloric acid, which not only compromises protein digestion, but also reduces IF secretion and therefore B12 absorption. For people with low hydrochloric acid production, supplementing hydrochloric acid (available with a doctor's prescription) may help digestion in the short term but in the long term will do nothing for IF secretion and B12 absorption. For minor digestive problems, eating bitter foods or taking bitter herbs may be a better solution because bitter substances stimulate the secretion of many digestive fluids in the stomach and the small intestine.

SECRET #2:

Under stress, the digestive system shuts down (the body shunts blood away from the digestive system and reduces digestive activity).

Our bodies simultaneously run two different nervous systems, the sympathetic and parasympathetic nervous systems. These two systems operate like a see-saw, with one or the other in the dominant position. The sympathetic nervous system primes us to react to stressful situations, triggering the "fight or flight" response in the body. During periods of relaxation, the body's parasympathetic nervous system predominates, encouraging tissue regeneration and repair. Consider the sympathetic nervous system "the general," ready to respond to danger at a moment's notice. Think of the parasympathetic nervous system as the masseuse or "the spa queen," thriving in a relaxed, nurturing environment.

For many people in today's culture the sympathetic nervous system predominates, with accompanying chronic low levels of norepinephrine (adrenaline) and other stress-related hormones. In earlier times, we would have expended norepinephrine and other hormones by moving our bodies – running from or fighting our attacker. Today, however, the "attacker" may be our boss, our landlady, or the IRS. No longer can we fight or run away; instead, we sit quietly and talk calmly. Our body, however, does not know the difference between a polar bear and an angry boss; the Generalissimo sympathetic nervous system responds the same way. Because we do not "use up" the stress related hormones by moving our bodies, we tend to live with chronic low levels of adrenaline in our system. Rarely does the body fully relax, completely activating the parasympathetic nervous system and therefore our body's repair and regeneration response.

When the sympathetic nervous system predominates, the body constricts the blood vessels that nourish the digestive system and dilates the blood vessels that feed the muscles, lungs, and heart. The body is preparing to use the muscles to fight or run away. During this emergency situation, digestive function is relatively unimportant. Chronic, low levels of stress hormones mean that the digestive system does not receive a full supply of blood. Peristalsis, the rhythmic

---

What this means for you:

The more relaxed you are, the better you will digest your food and the more nutrients you will absorb. Create a relaxed environment during meals.

118

movement of the digestive tract muscles, stops. Digestive secretions diminish, and if the digestive system shuts down for a period of time, food begins to putrefy. Clearly, with chronic levels of stress, our digestive system suffers.

Our digestive system functions best when we are relaxed. When the parasympathetic nervous system predominates, blood flow increases to the digestive tract, and more digestive juices flow. The stomach secretes more hydrochloric acid. The digestive tract also eliminates wastes more easily in this relaxed state.

Absorbing food

From the stomach, food moves into the small intestine. Another sphincter (the duodenal sphincter) separates the stomach and the small intestine, which is divided into three sections: the duodenum [doo-AH-den-um], jejunum [ju-JOON-um], and ileum [ILL-ee-um]. Most of the specialized digestive activity in the small intestine occurs in the duodenum, the first 12 inches of the small intestine. Only the duodenum, for example, absorbs vitamin B12. The pancreas secretes enzymes into the duodenum to digest carbohydrates, fats, and proteins. The gallbladder releases bile to break down fats and fat-based nutrients (e.g. vitamins A, D, and E). After stomach ulcers, the second most common site for ulcers is the duodenum. Knowing how many important digestive activities occur in the duodenum, you can understand how damaging an ulcer in this location would be. The majority of our food's nutrients enter the body through the three sections of the small intestine.

Eliminating waste

The food passes next into the large intestine, where water and certain nutrients are reabsorbed into the body. A third sphincter separates the small and large intestines. Remember that chronic low levels of the stress-related hormones slow peristalsis, the wavelike contractions in the digestive tract, and make us more prone to develop constipation. If the food waste tarries too long in the large intestine, waste products or "toxins" also re-enter the body. Ideally the food wastes remain no longer than 16 to 18 hours in the large intestine.

SECRET #3:
Food is your greatest ally.

When Hippocrates wrote his great treatises on health, most of his writings focused on food. "I saw this patient today, and I prescribed the following food . . ." was a common entry in his writings. To the average physician today, Hippocrates' work might seem trite or out-dated. What this scholar had discovered, however, was one of the major secrets of regaining and maintaining health: a healthy body requires carefully chosen food.

Patients often ask whether or not they need to take supplements. You can supplement nutrients in three

ways: with food, with a multi-vitamin and mineral supplement, and with single nutrients for specific deficiencies.

(Whole) food first

The best source of nutrients is food. By "food" I
mean substances that are as close as possible to their natural state. I have never seen a Twinkie tree, a Danish
pastry bush, or a Kool-Aid plant. I have read no reports
of Spam naturally occurring anywhere in the universe.
The more refined and processed our food, the more
nutrients we lose and the more health-defeating
substances we gain, such as preservatives, dyes, and
chemical stabilizers. Personally I am wary of ingesting
something that can last for months on a shelf. What
would that substance do inside me? Preservatives are a
boon for grocery stores but a hazard for our short and long
term health. Preservatives such as BHT, sodium nitrate,
and sodium nitrite break down into noxious toxic substances in our bodies. Our health suffers; only our
cadavers benefit. Funeral homes report that bodies last
longer than they did 50 years ago, probably as a result of
all of the preservatives in our food. I no longer consider
being "well preserved" a great compliment!

Eating whole foods guarantees that we receive more
nutrients and more fiber. Whole grains, for example,
have far more nutrients, particularly vitamin E and B
vitamins, and much more fiber than refined grains. Even
extractor juicers, touted for their health-enhancing properties, can diminish the value of whole foods. A cup of

extracted apple juice, for example, requires five fresh apples. The juice delivers a concentrated dose of sugar – yes, fructose or fruit sugar, but sugar nevertheless – and almost no fiber. You can easily drink a glass of apple juice, but could you eat five apples in one sitting? Not all juicers extract the fiber, however. Some juicers use the entire fruit or vegetable, including the nutrient- and fiber-rich pulp. These juicers, listed in Appendix B, can enhance absorption of nutrients.

SECRET #4:

Organically grown foods contain more nutrients than conventionally grown food.

According to California state law, "organic" means food grown without pesticides, insecticides, herbicides, or petroleum-based fertilizers. Certified organic farms have been "chemical-free" for at least three years. Recent studies demonstrate that organic foods have more nutrients than their conventionally grown counterparts.[1] Although organic foods may cost a bit more, they deliver more nutrients per serving, making up for the increased cost.

What this means for you:

Choose organic foods to maximize both your own and the Earth's health.

Organically grown foods also have the added benefit of supporting the health of our farmlands. Rain and irrigation water wash herbicides, insecticides, and fertilizers off agricultural lands and into our above and below ground water sources, killing aquatic life and poisoning our water supply. Conventional agriculture also exacts a heavy toll in terms of soil loss. Most conventional farms lose about 12 inches of topsoil per century. In contrast, a healthy prairie ecosystem generates one inch of topsoil every 1,000 years. In essence our agricultural system has "borrowed" over 12,000 years of soil in the last century. Supporting organic agriculture means increasing nutrients in our diet and improving the health of our farmlands.

Seasonal cycles, seasonal foods

When shopping for food, reach for locally grown produce rather than the exotic imports. Our bodies tend to respond best to foods grown in our local area which ripen in seasonal cycles that support our bodies' needs. Spring foods, for example, include many greens and bitter foods that improve liver and general digestive function. After a winter of eating heavier, fattier foods, the spring greens cleanse and reawaken the digestive system.

Spring greens give way to summer vegetables and berries. These water and nutrient-rich foods are easy to digest in the summer heat. During the light-filled summer months, we seem to draw more nourishment directly from the sun. With the light at its fullest, we tend to eat fewer complex carbohydrates and protein and instead emphasize more fresh, watery vegetables and fruits such as zucchini, string beans, peaches, lettuce, Swiss chard, and juicy berries.

As the summer progresses into autumn, the days shorten and the complex carbohydrate vegetables and grains ripen. Early autumn meals include corn, winter squash, beets, and other root vegetables. In temperate climates, winter meals rely on stored foods such as grains, apples, cabbage, and winter squash.

As the winter days shorten, we ingest sunlight stored in the form of grains, dried fruits, root vegetables, and other complex carbohydrates. Those who work outdoors require more calories and may increase vegetable oils as well as more complex carbohydrates in their diet. Traditionally the winter diet also included more meat and animal products such as milk, eggs, and cheese.

What this means for you:

Buy fresh, local food to reduce your food costs, save resources, and support your seasonal health needs.

"There's no place like home, there's no place like home."

Locally grown produce also supports the health of the environment. Local foods require less trucking, saving tons of fossil fuel per year. Local foods also require less spraying and preparation for market. Many of the imported fruits and vegetables are sprayed before leaving their country of origin. In addition, farmers in other countries spray exotic fruits and vegetables with chemicals long since outlawed in North America, including DDT. Bananas, for example, are one of the most heavily sprayed agricultural crops. If you must buy bananas, look for the organically grown, unsprayed varieties.

> **SECRET #5:**
> **Remember the big picture.**

Much of our current nutritional information focuses on specific nutrients and overlooks the importance of the Big Four food groups, or "macronutrients": protein, carbohydrates, fat, and water. If you make good choices in obtaining these four major nutrients, you will greatly increase your odds of ingesting the majority of the vitamins and minerals, or "micronutrients," you need as well.

Protein

How much protein should I be getting every day?

The answer depends on three factors: your stage in the lifecycle, your particular body needs, and the type of protein you are eating. Every nutrient in the body has a normal "window," what I call a "physiological amount" – the amount the body normally, naturally is used to seeing or producing. "Pharmacological" levels of a substance exceed the normal range, going far beyond the normal window.

The World Health Organization recommends 40 to 50 grams of protein a day for adult men and women, and 70 grams a day for pregnant and lactating women. People who do hard physical labor also require more protein, about 60 to 70

What this means for you:

A cup of lentils contains 17.9 grams of protein, a bagel has 6.0 grams, and a 4-ounce pork chop contains 27.6 grams of protein (along with a whopping 33 grams of fat).

grams per day. Most Americans, however, particularly meat eaters, consume far more than 40 to 50 grams of protein a day. Some stray into the pharmacological range of 100 to 150 grams of protein a day.

When we eat more protein than the body needs, the excess protein breaks down into sulfur-containing compounds called uric acid or urea. The kidneys must metabolize and excrete these breakdown products; hence a high protein diet puts extra strain on the kidneys.

Uric acid also increases the acidity of the blood stream. The body keeps careful tabs on the acid-alkaline balance (pH), and when the blood becomes too acidic, the body pulls calcium from the bones to buffer the increased acidity. We have known since 1920 that a high protein diet, particularly a high animal protein diet, causes more calcium to be excreted in the urine.[2] The amount of calcium dumped in the urine has the greatest impact on the health of our bones. Calcium loss effects bone density more dramatically than calcium intake or calcium absorption.[3] In other words, the amount of calcium we *lose* impacts bone health more dramatically than the amount of calcium we *absorb*. A high protein diet that exceeds the normal physiological window taxes our bones as well as our kidneys.

Animal and plant proteins have different effects on the body. Animal proteins consist largely of the amino acids methionine and cysteine, both of which break down into sulfate and hydrogen, which increase acidity in the body. Again, the

What this means for you:

For adults,

eat 40 to 50 grams

of protein per day.

Emphasize plant

sources of protein.

more acidic the body becomes, the more calcium is pulled from the bones. Plant proteins, in contrast, contain a very small percentage of these amino acids and do not have the same acidifying effect in the body.

Contrary to Mae West's declaration, "Too much of a good thing can be wonderful!", too much of even a good thing like protein can be problematic because doubling protein intake generally leads to a doubling of calcium loss as well.[4] Increases in plant protein, however, do not cause as much calcium excretion as increases in animal protein.

Fats and Oils

Does avoiding fat guarantee I will be healthy and lose weight?

On vacation in central Oregon, I wandered into a convenience store while waiting for our river-rafting trip to depart. Near the front counter I noticed a rack filled with candy. On closer inspection, I was shocked by the bright yellow stickers on the bags of neon-colored sweets: "Fat-Free!" At that moment I grasped the implications of our fanatical focus on fat. Most of us have been inculcated with the idea that "0 grams of fat" on the label means the food is healthy. Zero grams of fat, however, does not guarantee that the food is healthy, or that it will never be converted

What this means for you:

Consult a health care provider trained in nutrition about the optimal type and amount of protein for you, especially if you are considering completely eliminating animal protein.

to fat in the body! Most "health-oriented" consumers, swayed by conventional dietary wisdom, have identified fat as the demon. Avoiding the monstrous fat molecule, however, does not guarantee health or weight loss.

If we consume an excess of any food in our diet, the body converts surplus calories into fat. The "fat-free" candy, consisting mainly of sugar, artificial flavor, and food coloring, causes a quick rise in blood sugar. In response to high blood sugar levels, the body converts excess blood sugar into cholesterol and triglycerides (fats). Although fat was not listed on the label, highly sweetened foods definitely increase fat production in the body.

What this means for you:

If you want to reduce fat in your diet, reduce or eliminate simple sugars (e.g. white and brown sugar, honey, and corn syrup) as well.

Essential fatty acids

Despite its maligned media image, fat is one of several vital nutrients in our diet. We need fats for many important functions in the body. Cholesterol, for example, is the building block for all of our reproductive hormones. Cholesterol and fatty acids compose the cell wall of every cell in our body. We can manufacture several types of fat and cholesterol from other substances, but certain fats cannot be produced inside the body: linoleic acid and alpha-linolenic acid. These fats are referred to as "essential fatty acids" because our body cannot manufacture them, yet they are essential for normal, healthy bodies. We must provide these essential nutrients in our diet.

What's the difference between a fat and an oil?

I have a family member who insists that the margarine he liberally spreads on his toast " . . . is not fat." Despite numerous explanations, he is convinced that vegetable oils and fats are two completely different food groups. So what is the difference between a fat and an oil?

Not much. The main difference is the number of double bonds or "links" in their chains, and how solid or fluid the substances are at room temperature. Fats are made of glycerin, which has three "arms" with a chain of fatty acids attached to each arm. What do "chains" have to do with fats and oils? Nothing kinky, honestly. Fats and oils are made of long chains of carbons with hydrogen atoms attached. Think of them as long trains, with each carbon represented by a boxcar on the train. At the "engine" end of the train are three chains ending in "CH2" groups. At the caboose end are three – COOH groups, which makes that end acidic. This acidic tail explains why these long chains/trains are named "fatty acids."

Imagine the "hitches" between the boxcars as single or double connections, or "bonds" to use chemistry terms. The fewer the double hitches between the boxcars, the more solid the fat is at room temperature. Fats have only single "hitches" between the carbon atoms, which explains why they are solid at room temperature.

At the double hitches or "bonds," the carbon atoms are loosely attached to each other. Johanna Budwig, M.D., who has spent her life conducting pioneering research on fats and oils, describes these double hitches on the chain as " . . . fragile there, loose; it absorbs water easily – as if you were to fray a smooth silk thread in one place and then draw it through water. The frayed part absorbs water, or dye, more easily. In the same way, these fatty acid chains with their weak, unsaturated connections, form protein associations very easily. The fatty acids become water soluble through this association with protein."[5]

When we eat fats and oils, they travel across the intestines into the bloodstream. Remember that blood is a watery substance, and oil and water usually do not mix. These unsaturated fats, however, can become water soluble through their association with protein. Because these unsaturated fats with their double hitches between the boxcar can become water soluble, they are healthier forms of fat.

In contrast saturated fats cannot dissolve in the watery fluid of the blood. Hydrogenated oils, discussed in more detail below, are also insoluble in water. These solid fats "separate" in the blood, like oil and vinegar in salad dressing. Insoluble solid fats cannot circulate through the network of fine capillaries in the body; instead, they deposit along larger blood vessels walls, compromising circulation and promoting heart disease.

Olive oil is "mono-unsaturated" because it has only one double hitch on the carbon train. Olive oil is liquid at room temperature, but its single hitch ensures that the oil will solidify as it cools. The more double

What this means for you:

Emphasize unsaturated fats in your diet. Eliminate saturated fats and hydrogenated oils.

hitches on the train, the more fluid or "liquid" the train will be at room temperature and even cooler temperatures. "Polyunsaturated" oils have many hitches between the carbon boxcars and remain liquid even at low temperatures. Remember that multiple bonds also assure that the oil will associate with proteins and more easily dissolve in the blood.

Linoleic acid, one of the essential fatty acids, has two double bonds. Alpha-linolenic acid, the second essential fatty acid, has three double bonds. The first double bond on the linoleic molecule is at the sixth carbon (boxcar on the train), which is why linoleic acid is called an "omega-6" fatty acid. For alpha-linolenic acid, the first double bond is at the third carbon, which explains its designation as an "omega-3" fatty acid.

Most nutrition experts recommend that we maintain a ratio of three to four times more linoleic acid than alpha-linolenic acid (3:1 or 4:1 ratio). Eating the Standard American Diet (SAD), nutritionists estimate most Americans consume 20 *times* more linoleic than alpha-linolenic acid (20:1 ratio). That means most people eat five to seven times more linoleic acid than they need.

In normal, "physiological" amounts, linoleic essential fatty acid reduces inflammatory activity in the body. Too much of even "good" linoleic fatty acid, however, can have the opposite effect and boost inflammatory reactions. Re-establishing a

What this means for you:

Unsaturated fats become water soluble and "dissolve" in the blood when associated with protein. In contrast, insoluble saturated fats and hydrogenated oils thicken the blood, deposit along blood vessel walls, and promote heart disease.

What this means for you:

Too much of even a "good" oil can increase inflammatory conditions in the body.

normal ratio of essential fatty acids, i.e. reducing linoleic and increasing alpha-linolenic acid, can improve several conditions, including rheumatoid arthritis, atherosclerosis, high blood pressure, and possibly even cancer.

Fish oils are rich in the "good" omega-3 and omega-6 fatty acids. Studies demonstrate that supplementing fish oils can decrease blood pressure and lower cholesterol levels.[6] Certain plant oils also contain high amounts of omega-3 and omega-6 fatty acids. Plant oils containing alpha-linolenic acid (listed below) may be healthier sources of omega-3 and omega-6 fatty acids than fish oils which tend to become rancid during the manufacturing process. Most fish oils also cost more than plant oils.

To establish a normal ratio of essential fatty acids, emphasize alpha-linolenic fatty acids in the diet. Remember that we need both essential fatty acids in the diet in small amounts.

Saturated fats (minimize or eliminate these):
- Animal fat, especially high in red meats
- Palm oil

Hydrogenated oils (eliminate these)
- Margarine
- Vegetable shortening
- Any packaged foods containing "hydrogenated vegetable oil"

Oils rich in linoleic essential fatty acid
(small amounts of these):

- Evening primrose oil
- Black currant seed oil
- Borage oil
- Canola
- Soy
- Corn
- Safflower
- DHA (fish oil)

Oils rich in alpha-linolenic essential fatty acid
(emphasize these):

- EPA (fish oil)
- Flaxseed oil (the richest natural source of
  omega-3 fatty acids)

Quality is as important as quantity of fat

Choose oils and fats as close as possible to their
natural state. Most margarines are made with altered fats
called "*trans* fatty acids." Remember chemistry class and
those noxious fumes you generated under the laboratory
hood? One of the few concepts from organic chemistry
that still serves me is the understanding of *cis* and
trans molecular formations, which describe the three-
dimensional structure of the molecule. Normally the
hydrogen atoms attached to carbon in a fat molecule are
in the same plane, on the same "side" of the molecule
(*cis* formation). Think of the train with hydrogen atoms
attached to the same side of the boxcar. Heating fat
molecules and adding hydrogen atoms changes the
molecular structure. These altered *trans* fatty acids have
hydrogen molecules attached on opposite sides of

the molecule, across from (*trans*) each other.

Over-heating "good" polyunsaturated oil breaks the "double hitches" between the carbon boxcars, and hydrogen atoms fill the missing gaps. Remember that the fewer the "hitches" or bonds, the more solid the oil is at room temperature. The added hydrogen atoms bond on the opposite (*trans*) side of the boxcar, which further stabilizes the molecule. In essence, heating and hydrogenating vegetable oils changes them from "good" poly-unsaturated oil to "bad" saturated fats.

Think about the difference between a baked and a fried potato. The baked potato remains soft. The fried potato becomes "crispy," or more solid. At high temperatures, the "good" vegetable oil used to fry the potato transforms into a *trans* fatty acid, causing the crispier, more solid texture. The fried food may taste good, but we lose the beneficial features of the polyunsaturated vegetable oil and gain the health destroying effects of *trans* fatty acids.

These *trans* fatty acids became more widely available with the introduction of margarine to replace butter, a scarce commodity during the Great Depression of the 1930s. After WWII, food manufacturers began to incorporate these altered oils in processed foods such as bakery products, peanut butter, and shortening. Today only the most vigilant can completely avoid *trans* fatty acids.

Only now are we beginning to understand the long-term effects of consuming *trans* fatty acids. A study

---

What this means for you:

For bread, butter is a better choice than margarine, and olive oil is better yet – adopt the Italian custom of dipping bread in fresh olive oil.

published in *Lancet*, the premier British medical journal, demonstrated that women eating a diet high in *trans* fatty acids (e.g. margarine, vegetable shortening, and fried foods) have much higher risk of developing coronary heart disease.[7] In contrast, people eating a "Mediterranean" diet, high in fresh vegetables, fruits, fish, and olive oil, have significantly lower risk of heart disease.[8]

Remember that fatty acids compose the cell wall of every cell in our body. The increased incidence of many chronic diseases may be a side effect of incorporating these altered fats, e.g. *trans* fatty acids and hydrogenated oils, into our cell walls.

How much fat do I need in my diet?

In a previous section we discussed the ideal ratio of essential fatty acids. Now let's look at the recommended quantity of fat in the diet. Usually dietary recommendations suggest the ideal percentage of calories derived from fat rather than a specific amount. For people consuming a traditional Asian diet, about 10 percent of their calories come from fat. To achieve this truly low fat diet means cooking with little or no oil. The vast majority of fat on a 10 percent fat diet naturally occurs in the foods. Whole grains, for example, contain tiny amounts of oil, as do vegetables. Nuts and seeds contain higher amounts of naturally occurring oils. The low fat content of the Asian diet may account for lower breast and colon cancer rates as well as a host of other chronic diseases.

In contrast to the Asian diet, most North Americans derive a prodigious 40 to 50 percent of their calories from fat!

What kinds of oils should I choose?

Remember that the type of fat you eat may be as important as the quantity. Someone may jubilantly report that they have reduced their fat consumption to 20 percent of their daily calories, but if the majority of that fat is from hydrogenated margarine, they have little reason to celebrate.

Aim for a diet with 10 to 15 percent of your calories derived from fats. Ideally those fats would be naturally occurring oils in the food you eat, supplemented with olive oil for cooking and small amounts of flaxseed or other cold-pressed oils for salad dressings.

Nuts and seeds are good sources of natural oils. You need only a small quantity – a handful, or a couple of tablespoons of a seed or nut – to fulfill your daily needs for oil. Make sure you are eating fresh nuts and seeds. All oils, even naturally occurring oils, may become oxidized, or "rancid." Once fat or oil oxidizes, it does more harm than good in the body.

An "oxidized" food contains free oxygen, which acts as a "free radical" in the body. No, this is not a flashback from the Seventies – a "free radical" is a substance with oxygen attached. Obviously we need oxygen in the air we breathe to nourish every cell in the body. Too much oxygen, or oxygen in the wrong place, however, can damage the body. The body keeps very tight control over oxygen absorption and transport in the body. Carbon quickly combines with oxygen waste to form CO2, carbon dioxide. Other substances, known as "antioxidants," also combine with and neutralize oxygen. If oxygen had free reign in the body with no regulation whatsoever, oxygen would "oxidize," or damage, the cells in our body.

Eating rancid oils is an easy way to ingest a host of "free radicals." The body then has to expend a lot of nutrients and energy to chase down and attach something to those free-ranging oxygen molecules. If our body has to allocate many of its resources to remedy the side effects of rancid food, we have less energy to take care of other important business, like nourishing and repairing cells.

Oils may go rancid even before they have the characteristic stale, bitter smell. If a jar of nuts or seeds smells rancid, they have long since passed the healthful eating stage. Any food, for that matter, that smells rancid is a good candidate for the compost heap or the trash can. "Wasting" rancid food by tossing it in the garbage is a better choice than trashing the body with a host of free radicals.

The same wisdom holds true for oils. If oil smells stale, it has long since become rancid. Discard these oils immediately. You can increase the longevity of oils by keeping them in a cool, dark place, e.g. in the refrigerator. Even olive oil should be refrigerated. If refrigerated olive oil hardens,

What this means for you:

Throw away oil, nuts, or seeds that smell stale or rancid.

simply place the bottle in a bowl of warm water for a few minutes, and the oil will melt to liquid again.

Most manufacturers extract oils from nuts or seeds with chemicals and heat. Remember that heat changes the "hitches on the boxcars," the configuration of the oil molecule. Cold-pressed oils are a better choice than conventionally extracted oils. These cold-pressed oils may cost a bit more, but they are worth the savings in the free radical clean up the body has to do.

What this means for you:

Choose cold-pressed oils, and store them in the refrigerator. Even olive oil should be kept in the refrigerator.

Exposing the "fake" fat

Olestra™, Procter and Gamble's new alternative to oil, cannot be absorbed in the digestive tract. "Eureka!" you may think. "All the wonderful taste of fat without the calories!" Unfortunately Olestra™ quickly exits the digestive tract along with other oil-soluble nutrients like vitamins A, E, and D. Lycopene is one the strongest anti-oxidants known. One serving of Olestra™ causes a 60 percent drop in lycopene absorption. Focus on naturally occurring oils, not high tech substitutes that strip the body of vital nutrients.

CARBOHYDRATES

SECRET #6: **Complex carbohydrates can help reduce weight.**

Do you remember the diets of the late 70s that emphasized protein and recommended completely eliminating carbohydrates? Most of the books portrayed carbohydrates as demonic fat builders, sure to add unsightly pounds with the merest morsel.

Simple carbohydrates and the blood sugar roller coaster

Most of these tomes, however, overlooked the difference between simple and complex carbohydrates. Simple carbohydrates include milled flours and concentrated sugars – what I call "the white wonders," e.g. white flour, white rice, and white sugar. These simple carbohydrates quickly break down in the digestive tract and enter the blood stream like white lightening. Blood sugar levels skyrocket, and the pancreas goes on red alert, dumping insulin into the blood stream to normalize blood sugar levels. Initially the pancreas over-reacts, dumping too much insulin into the blood stream. Within 30 to 45 minutes blood sugar plummets, often to levels lower than before eating the simple carbohydrate. The sudden drop in sugar may lead to headaches, fatigue, poor concentration, and grumpiness. "Oooh," you groan,

"I just need another one of those sticky buns and a cup of coffee. Then I'll be able to tackle this report." You eat the pastry, drink the coffee, and blood sugar quickly skyrockets. You strap yourself in for the next roller coaster ride.

Many people ride this blood sugar roller coaster all day long. No wonder people arrive home at the end of the day too exhausted to do more than eat (usually another round of simple carbohydrates like white spaghetti, red wine, white bread, and some nutrient-free iceberg lettuce) and watch television.

Complex carbohydrates

Complex carbohydrates are grains, legumes, root vegetables, and winter squashes that are as close as possible to their natural state. Complex carbohydrates contain far more nutrients than their stripped simple carbohydrate counterparts. In addition, the complex carbohydrates have lots of both soluble and insoluble fiber. Insoluble fibers, such as wheat bran, make you feel full with fewer calories and also "sweep" the intestines as they move through the digestive tract. Water-soluble fiber, such as oat bran, increases satiety [sah-TIE-it-ee] (the full sensation in the stomach), reduces the uptake of oils, slows the absorption of sugars, and lubricates the digestive tract.

Satiety is an important signal for the hunger center in the brain. Until a certain bulk of food stretches the stomach, we still feel hungry. Remember that a gram of fat or oil contains nine calories. In contrast, proteins and carbohydrates contain three calories per gram.

Imagine eating a large order of French fries, a cheeseburger, and a 12-ounce soft drink. You could easily fit that amount of food in your stomach. This meal includes lots of fat (French fries, beef burger, cheese, mayonnaise – 41 grams of fat total), some protein, and simple carbohydrates (sugar in the soda and white flour in the bun). The total calorie count is 902 calories (not including dessert). You probably would have no problem fitting in another order of French fries and a dessert.

To get the same number of calories from complex carbohydrates, vegetables, and protein, you would have to eat:

> 2 ears of fresh corn, steamed
> 1 cup of steamed broccoli
> 1 cup of spinach
> 1 hard boiled egg
> 1 3-inch whole wheat bagel
> 2 medium apples
> 2 medium baked potatoes (with no butter or
>   sour cream)

Total calorie count: 850 calories

If you absolutely had to eat some fat, one tablespoon of butter would add an additional 100 calories for a total of 950 calories.

Few people could eat this much food at one sitting!

Eating complex carbohydrates means obtaining more nutrients, more fiber, and fewer calories

What this means for you:

You can eat more food and still lose weight if you focus mainly on complex carbohydrates, fruits, and vegetables.

in the same sized serving of food. You literally can eat more and still lose weight by eating mainly complex carbohydrates, fruits, and vegetables.

SECRET #7:

Some "natural," unprocessed foods cause sharp peaks and drops in blood sugar levels.

Certain foods, even in their unprocessed, natural state, can dramatically increase blood sugar levels. The "glycemic index" measures the blood sugar response to a variety of foods. Those foods with a "high" glycemic index cause a quick increase in blood sugar levels, while "low" glycemic index foods help maintain lower, steadier blood sugar levels. Beans, for example, have a low glycemic index, helping to maintain steady blood sugar levels over several hours. For those suffering with type II diabetes or hypoglycemia (low blood sugar), a breakfast of black beans and tortillas maintains steady blood sugar levels for three to four hours. A food's ability to increase blood sugar is not always directly related to the number of calories it contains. Carrots, the quintessential dieter's companion, have a very high glycemic index, causing a sharp rise in blood sugar levels.

WATER

Healing waters

Water comprises about 70 percent of the human body; similarly, water covers over 70 percent of the Earth's surface. The amount of sodium in our blood reflects the ocean's salinity. In essence we carry the ocean within ourselves, harboring the same salinity in our blood as the oceanic "life blood" of the planet. In order to sustain this oceanic salinity, our bodies maintain a delicate balance between holding and excreting water. Many factors can alter the body's water metabolism, including diet, kidney function, cardiovascular health, digestion, and hormone balance.

Diet has a major impact on water metabolism, contributing to either dehydration or water retention. Certain foods have a diuretic effect, causing water loss, while others encourage the body to hold water, leading to bloating and water retention. One cup of a caffeinated beverage, for example, causes a loss of two cups of fluid. Alcohol also acts as a diuretic in the body. After over-indulging, dehydration contributes to the characteristic "hangover." In April 1990 *Business Magazine* in Canada reported that millions of North Americans consume two-thirds of their water from coffee. Several million more imbibe one-third or more of their water in the form of beer. That means that by the end of the day, most North Americans have created a water deficit in the body.

Not drinking enough fluid ironically may cause water

retention. Decreased fluid means increased break down products, or "toxins," that the body cannot eliminate through the kidneys, so the body holds water to try to dilute these toxic products. The build up of metabolic waste products can lead to fatigue, foggy thinking, irritability, headaches, and a host of other symptoms.

Water quality

Increasing water consumption can improve your energy, mental alertness, and general well being. Most municipal water sources in North America, however, deliver chemically treated water that may cause more harm than good. Most municipalities add chlorine to the drinking water to kill bacteria and other organisms. Chlorine serves an important function in delivering water to our homes; however, ingesting chlorine destroys many nutrients, particularly the B vitamins, and increases xeno-estrogen activity in the body. "Xeno" means foreign, so "xenoestrogens" are foreign substances that have estrogen-like activity in the body. Estrogen stimulates growth, particularly in cells of the breasts, testes, and uterus. Too much estrogen activity can increase the risk of reproductive cancers in both men and women.

Plastics can release chemicals that have xeno-estrogen effects in the body. Drinking water stored in plastic bottles may contain chemicals that have migrated into the water, especially if the plastic container is heated

What this means for you:

For optimum health, drink at least eight 8-ounce glasses of water a day (or two liters for the metric world).

because most plastics destabilize when exposed to heat. Leaving a plastic water bottle in the back of the car on a sunny day, for example, is a great way to encourage plastic to migrate into the water. Drinking hot beverages in plastic or Styrofoam cups also encourages plastic migration. Plastic water pipes, particularly those made of PVC, can leach chemicals into the water.

Check the bottom of your plastic bottles. One form of plastic, marked with the number seven, is much more stable and less likely to migrate into the water. Many health food stores now carry half-gallon water containers made with number seven plastic.

Water sources also may be polluted with chemicals from agricultural run-off and industrial effluents. In some areas giardia and other water-borne microorganisms are becoming commonplace in the drinking water supply. Some states are considering requiring water filters in all homes because the local water boards can no longer guarantee delivery of safe drinking water.

Even homeowners with their own water source, such as a spring or well, need to be cautious. Toxic chemical dumps, chemical spills, and agricultural run off may contaminate ground water. If you live near a national forest, contact the local forestry office to ask about spraying in your area. The U.S. Forest Service periodically sprays to eliminate (or prevent) insect plagues.

What this means for you:

Choose water containers made with number seven plastic. Heat water in glass, metal, or ceramic containers, and drink hot fluids from a ceramic cup.

Don't wait for your local water board to notify you about contaminants in your water supply. The Environmental Protection Agency (EPA) sets "safe" levels of many contaminants to minimize (not avoid) deaths, not to maximize health. Consider having your water tested. Contact your local water board for testing information. Unless you live in a pristine out-post of modern "civilization," you probably would benefit from installing a water filter for both drinking and bathing water. Choose one that filters chlorine, petrochemicals, heavy metals, bacteria, and other organisms. Many of the newer filters pass water through several media to filter different types of pollutants.

What this means for you:

A good water filter can dramatically improve water quality.

Water filters are wonderful allies to improve the quality of our water. Water filters, however, only address symptoms. They improve the quality of the water coming from the faucet, but they do nothing for the health of the water in our larger environment. In the long run, the best remedy would be to make choices that support the health of our water supply, e.g. carefully considering the impact of the chemicals we us in our environment, how we dispose of wastes, and how much water we use. The more water we use, the more water the local water board must process before it can be returned to our homes or local streams and rivers.

MICRONUTRIENTS

Micronutrients include vitamins and minerals, substances vital to our health that we need in small quantities. You can find many resources that discuss the individual functions of the vitamins and minerals. In this section I want to approach the micronutrients from a broader view.

Our bodies need all of the micronutrients to function optimally. Foods contain a combination of vitamins and minerals. All of the metabolic pathways in our bodies require particular vitamins and/or minerals, which act as catalysts or regulators of these pathways. Nutrients were meant to work in combination with one another.

Consider the nutrient calcium, for example. Many menopausal women concerned about bone health ask, "How much calcium should I take?"

"What other nutrients are you taking?" is my reply. Calcium alone cannot build strong bones. Bone health depends on calcium, magnesium, all of the other minerals, and several vitamins as well. How often have you walked in a field and tripped over a chunk of calcium lying on the ground? You will almost never find one mineral by itself because the molecular configuration guarantees that the mineral must be bound to another substance, usually another mineral. Similarly, our bodies require the full spectrum of vitamins and minerals to function optimally. In fact, supplementing a large quantity of a single nutrient may actually inhibit the absorption or function of another nutrient. Supplementing large amounts of calcium, for example, drives down magnesium supplies in the body. Calcium and magnesium compete for absorption in the intestines. Normally foods

What this means for you:

A supplement cannot take the place of eating whole, fresh foods.

containing calcium also contain magnesium, so the body absorbs some of each nutrient.

We have a normal range or "window" for every substance in the body. We can have problems if we step outside the window, taking either too much or too little of that substance into the body. We call less than the normal window a "deficiency." "Physiological" amounts fall within the normal range and provide what the body normally, naturally utilizes. Going beyond the window, we enter "pharmacological" levels which exceed the normal, natural amounts the body needs. Even with vital nutrients like protein or calcium, we run into problems when we stray outside the physiological window for that substance.

Remember that food is the best source of nutrients. Organic foods contain more nutrients than conventionally grown food, so you can increase micronutrients in your diet by choosing organic foods. Conventional agricultural practices strip the soil of nutrients and add little or no humus back to the soil. As the soil quality deteriorates, so does the nutritional value of our foods.

Remember that a good multi-vitamin and mineral supplement can enhance, but not take the place of, a good diet. Each body is different, and some people may need larger quantities of a particular substance. Working with a well-trained health care provider can maximize the effectiveness of the supplements you take. Taking

---

What this means for you:

Consider taking a good multi-vitamin and mineral supplement, particularly if you live in a polluted environment and do not eat regular meals.

---

fistfuls of supplements willy nilly may waste your money and possibly even undermine your health.

> **SECRET #8:**
> **One person's food may be another**
> **person's poison.**

As I child I got sick like clockwork every six weeks, starting from the time I was an infant. My mother breast-fed me for six weeks, so I had a good start. From six weeks on, however, I would get sick every six weeks, usually with an ear infection, nasty upper respiratory infection, or bronchitis. I spent a lot of my childhood sick and frustrated. When I was about 10 or 11 years old I began to read books about health. I practiced yoga and tried adding certain "healthy" foods to my diet. Fortunately my family already had a fairly healthy diet, including lots of vegetables from our backyard organic garden.

During the winter of my 12th year, I caught a bad cold that settled into my lungs. I expelled prodigious amounts of green phlegm for over three months. I was exhausted and weary of being sick. When my mother took me to the doctor for the third or fourth round of antibiotics, she finally confronted the physician.

"I don't understand this," said my mother, looking the doctor squarely in the eye. "She eats a good diet – whole grain bread, very little sugar, lots of fruits and vegetables. She exercises, sleeps enough, and takes good care of herself. Why won't this bronchitis go away?"

The doctor curled his forefinger above his chin and crossed the other arm across his chest. He thought for a few moments before answering.

"Well," he said ponderously, "I could refer you to an EENT specialist, someone who could see if she has something going on in her sinuses or her respiratory system in general. You can call and make an appointment – you'll probably have to wait a few weeks to get in. That's about all I can suggest."

Thanks to my mother's insistence, I did get an appointment with the specialist. He immediately suspected food or inhalant allergies and referred me for allergy testing. I endured the skin prick tests for inhalant allergies and discovered I was sensitive to ragweed. The blood test for food allergies revealed "mild" allergies to eggs, tomatoes, oranges, yeast, and corn.

Initially I wondered what I would eat. Corn is ubiquitous in the American diet, particularly in any kind of packaged food. Many foods contain eggs and/or lecithin. Unless the label specified "soy lecithin," I had to assume the lecithin came from eggs. I did manage to eliminate the foods from my diet, not an easy task for a teenager. I discovered that many of the "healthy" foods I had been eating were not healthy for me. Whole grain breads were an improvement over Wonder Bread, but they still contained yeast, one of my food allergens. Pizza parties, the mainstay of many teenagers' social lives, were a nightmare for me. I would eat the mushrooms on the pizza and leave the rest for my friends.

The hard work changing my diet paid off quickly, however. Within 14 days the three-month bout of bronchitis resolved. My energy skyrocketed. I no longer felt like I was always on the edge of catching a cold. The incessant colds became less frequent. In high school I never missed a day of school because of illness.

During the first few months after discovering the food allergies, I learned a whole new way of cooking. At 13 I was already a fairly proficient cook and soon learned how to cook whole grains and bake unleavened breads. I read, learned, cooked, and began to feel better and better. The learning process was a relief, not a chore, because my health was improving in dramatic ways.

From my own experience I know that the optimal food for one person may be poison for another. The recommended "healthy" foods won't help Suzie or Johnny if they are allergic to those foods. After eating a food you are allergic to, the body mobilizes the immune system to react to the food as if it were a foreign invader like a bacteria or virus. The immune system expends its energy "fighting" this allergen-invader, expending its resources so that the immune system has less energy to address other challenges.

By "allergies" I mean specific immune system mediated reactions in the body. We may also react to foods in ways that do not involve the immune system, in which case the reactions are referred to as "food sensitivities."

Our body has two different types of immune system responses to allergens. Immuneglobulin E (IgE) mediated reactions are classic allergic reactions that involve hives, itching, and in severe circumstances, swelling of the throat and bronchi. If the swelling is extreme, a severe IgE allergic reaction can kill you. This severe "anaphylactic" reaction can happen only with the second or later exposure to a substance. The first exposure sensitizes the immune system, and the second exposure elicits the full immune response. The first bee sting, for example, cannot cause an anaphylactic reaction, but the second episode could because the immune system is primed to react. Most people know if they have a severe IgE reaction to a particular substance – the symptoms are simply too dramatic to ignore.

Immuneglobulin G (IgG) allergic reactions are less obvious and therefore often go undetected. IgG reactions may occur from a few hours to four days after eating the allergen. The time delay can make these allergies difficult if not impossible to detect.

How do I know if I have food allergies or sensitivities?

Checking the list of symptoms below can provide some clues as to whether or not you suffer from food allergies. Keep in mind, though, that many of these symptoms can be related to a wide variety of conditions, not just food allergies. If you regularly have several of these symptoms, you may be a good candidate for food allergy or food sensitivity testing:

- Headaches
- Heartburn
- Abdominal bloating

- Sneezing
- Itchy skin
- Itching around the anus
- Dark circles under the eyes ("allergic shiners")
- Hyperactivity in children
- Mood swings
- Irritability
- Ear infections
- Poor memory
- Lack of concentration
- Nasal stuffiness
- Sinus pain
- Coughing
- Frequent colds or flu
- Flu-like symptoms
- Joint pain
- Fatigue
- Hypoglycemia (low blood sugar)

The following tests can help determine whether or not you have food allergies or sensitivities:
- Elimination diet: considered the "gold standard" among many physicians and nutritionists, the elimination diet requires fasting or following a limited, hypoallergenic diet for a few days, then adding foods one at a time and watching how the body reacts. The elimination diet pinpoints the foods you react to as well as the specific reactions associated with those foods. You still may miss some delayed sensitivity reactions, however.

- Blood tests: the RAST test is the best of the blood tests now available for detecting IgE and IgG (immediate and delayed) allergies. RAST mostly has replaced cytotoxic blood tests, an earlier approach to food allergy testing.

- VEGA (electroacupuncture according to Vole): this testing method uses a machine that creates an electrical circuit between a specific point on the body (usually around the nail bed of one of the fingers) and a particular food substance. The machine passes a very low voltage of current through the circuit and measures any change in the strength of the current. Foods that diminish the electrical current are eliminated or rotated in the diet. This testing method does not detect food "allergies," because the system is not checking IgE and IgG immune system reactions. Instead the VEGA system checks for food "sensitivities."

- Muscle testing or "reflexology": Like the VEGA test, muscle testing detects food sensitivities, not allergies. The practitioner asks the patient to resist while s/he presses down on the patient's arm (or sometimes foot). After establishing a baseline "strength," the practitioner asks the patient to hold a food or other substance, usually over the center of the chest or the solar plexus. Again, the practitioner asks the patient to "resist" the downward pressure. If the muscle increases in strength, the food is "strengthening" the body. If the muscle weakens, the food must be "weakening" the body. The effectiveness of this testing method varies radically with the practitioner's ability. I personally would not recommend relying on this method as the sole means of detecting food allergies or sensitivities.

How do food allergies develop?

The truth is that medical science does not have a clear, easy answer for why people develop or are born with food allergies. Medical science has developed several theories about how food allergies develop, each of which may provide some clues: leaky gut syndrome, genetic predisposition, pesticides on foods, hybridized plants, and borderline poisonous foods.

Leaky gut syndrome: Considered a "fringe" theory a decade ago, many internists and gastroenterologists now consider this a likely explanation for food allergies and a host of other digestive problems. A decade ago, most physicians assumed the digestive tract would break down any food into basic components – proteins automatically digested to amino acids, oils to free fatty acids, fruits and vegetables to fructose, vitamins, and minerals. Medical researchers assumed that the digestive tract always remained healthy. We had iron stomachs and titanium intestines – nothing could phase these digestive organs. Many physicians also assumed that diet had no effect whatsoever on health. I'm not sure where they thought the nutrients in a person's body came from, but food was not an important source.

Slowly the general medical wisdom is shifting. More

physicians now recognize that certain foods supply vital nutrients for the body while other foods may damage the lining of the intestines and deliver health destroying substances to the body. Highly processed, fiber deficient foods move slowly in the digestive tract. Saturated fats and animal proteins also move sluggishly in the digestive tract. Slow moving food begins to putrefy, and the mucosa, or lining, of the intestine suffers. Initially the gut lining becomes inflamed. Later, if the insults continue, the lining becomes chronically inflamed, and the cells lose their integrity. The tight connections between the intestinal cells called "gap junctions" deteriorate. Instead of meeting a carefully controlled gate (gap junction), the digested food meanders through a broken fence. No longer able to maintain a carefully controlled border, the intestinal lining becomes "leaky," allowing large food particles to pass through the "gates" or gap junctions that normally would have stopped them.

What this means for you:

A chronically irritated digestive tract increases your chances of developing food allergies.

When these large food particles enter the blood stream, the immune system may view them as foreign invaders. Accustomed to seeing food components like amino acids and free fatty acids, these large particles may trigger a "red alert" and eventually cause the immune system to tag these food particles as "invaders," or in medical terms "allergens." When the large particles enter the blood stream, the immune system mounts an attack on the invader, causing a set of allergic symptoms specific to that food in that individual.

Genetic predisposition: Another theory suggests that our bodies adapted to the foods commonly eaten during our evolution; hence, foods from distant lands are not familiar to our digestive tract or our immune system. Those of northern European ancestry, for example, until very recently have had little exposure to tropical fruits. If someone moved from Ireland to northern Australia, the body might develop allergies to the new foods indigenous to the tropics. The genetic theory holds that our digestive system does not adapt to new circumstances as quickly as our bodies can move. The genetic material is a slower-moving, more stable encoding system. Our bodies may require several generations to adapt to new food sources.

Pesticides on foods and plant hybrids: I include these two together because both relate to modern agricultural practices. Two of the most common food allergens in the United States are corn and soybeans. Most farmers heavily spray both of these crops with petrochemical insecticides and pesticides. Some nutritionists suggest that "allergic" reactions result from the toxic chemicals sprayed on the plants, not because of the plants themselves.

In the last century we have learned to hybridize plants, to cross two genetically similar "parents" to produce new offspring called "hybrids." The seeds gathered and replanted from these hybrid creations revert to the parent stock. Another theory, similar to the "genetic predisposition" hypothesis, is that our bodies do not recognize these new hybrid creations as "food." Indeed, researchers created many plant hybrids with factors other than nutrition in mind – behold the square tomato, genetically engineered to fit more economically into tomato packing boxes. And tomatoes bring us to the last theory . . . .

Borderline poisonous foods: Tomatoes are part of the genus *Solonaceae,* commonly known as the nightshade family. Thornton Wilder, in his play *Our Town,* satirizes our uncertainty about the safety of eating plants from the nightshade family. Almost a century later, researchers continue to debate whether or not the nightshades truly are edible plants. Some of the species definitely are out of bounds, e.g. the deadly nightshade. Others linger in our diets, passing in and out of vogue according to the research of the times. The (debatably) edible nightshades include tomatoes, potatoes, eggplants, and peppers. The edible nightshades have been implicated in causing or exacerbating osteoarthritis, but they seem to have little effect on rheumatoid arthritis. The recent nutritional craze over anti-oxidants, however, favors the consumption of tomatoes which contain high amounts of lycopene, a substance known to have stronger antioxidant activity than vitamin E.

Are allergies a permanent condition?

We have no definitive answer about what causes food allergies (probably multiple factors contribute), and we also have no definitive "cure" for food allergies. Researchers and clinicians have developed many approaches to address allergic symptoms (e.g. shots or diluted oral doses of the allergens), but few methods touch the root of the problem. For those suffering with "leaky gut syndrome," rebuilding the intestinal lining and restoring the digestive system to health may reduce or eliminate allergic reactions. Dr. Nampudripad has developed her own system to "eliminate" allergies that integrates muscle testing and acupuncture (Nampudripad's Allergy Elimination Technique, NAET). As mentioned above, the effectiveness of this system relies on the practitioner's reflexology skills.

Choosing organic, non-hybridized foods also may reduce allergic symptoms. A friend sensitive to dairy products traveling in Germany noted that German milk and cheese, taken from cows raised sans hormones and antibiotics, did not bother her digestive system. Remember that some "allergies" may in fact be reactions to chemicals sprayed on the food, or the new hybrid strains that are foreign to our digestive system. You can increase nutrients in your diet and minimize allergic tendencies by choosing organic foods.

SECRET #9:
How to have terrible indigestion in one easy meal.

Prepare a beautiful meal with fresh organic vegetables, trout caught from a pure mountain stream, and wild rice. Carry your delicious meal to the table and turn on the television to watch the evening news. As you eat, watch the President or some other legislator trying to squirm out of a ream of new allegations. Ponder your rapidly shrinking investments as you watch the stock market report flicker on the screen. Cringe as soldiers dodge bullets in a war torn province and gasp at the report of horrific child abuse in your neighborhood.

By the end of the meal, you may have chewed a total of fifty times. Your heart is shredded and your nervous system is on red alert. Remember that the sympathetic nervous system does not differentiate between a bear market and a bear in the woods. The body prepares to fight or flee, dumping adrenaline and other hormones into the bloodstream. The heart speeds up and blood rushes into the muscles . . . while you sit rooted to the chair. The body reduces blood flow to the internal organs, precisely when you need circulation in the digestive organs to break down and absorb food. Unfortunately you may absorb few of the nutrients from the wonderful meal.

You can further guarantee indigestion by substituting animal meat smothered with fat-dripping gravy for the fish, soaking up the gravy with white bread, and trading a baked potato swimming with margarine for the wild rice. Avoid anything that looks remotely green (unless you are searching for Jell-O™ in the refrigerator). Eat a large bowl of premium ice cream with maximum milk fat for dessert.

Another quick way to develop indigestion is to eat while trying to accomplish other tasks. Many people, myself included, eat their lunch (if they eat at all) while careening along the freeway, driving with one hand and

What this means for you:

Sit down while eating rather than gulping food while driving 70 miles an hour. Save arguments or studies for another time.

alternately biting a sandwich and dialing a cell phone with the other. To maximize the value of your food, consider sitting still while eating. Create a relaxed environment. Play soothing music and choose a beautiful place setting. The digestive system functions best when the body is relaxed. Consider putting aside even reading materials while you eat. In Chinese medicine, particular organs or body systems are related to certain emotions. Each organ has a primary emotion that strengthens and one that weakens that organ's function. Joy, for example, strengthens the heart while sadness weakens it. From Chinese medical perspective, too much thinking or worrying disrupts the function of the digestive organs. No wonder students often suffer from digestive upsets. Students spend the majority of their time worrying about exams, thinking, and studying, including while they are eating!

SECRET #10:
Chew your food.

How often did your mother or father roll their eyes and remind you to chew your food? Well, they were right. Funny how wise our parents become as we grow older – when did they become so smart? This simple bit of advice can save hundreds of dollars in over-the-counter medications and trips to the doctor's office.

Remember that digestion begins in the mouth. As you chew food, you begin the break down

What this means for you:

Chew your drink and drink your food.

process making a larger surface area available to extract more nutrients from the food. In addition, chewing mixes the food with saliva which contains amylase, an enzyme that begins the digestion of carbohydrates.

SECRET #11:
Choose fresh foods.

As mentioned earlier, food is your greatest ally, and fresh food is the best of all. I am blessed with a large vegetable garden in my back yard, and nothing compares with the flavor of steamed greens picked 15 minutes earlier from the garden. The fresher your food, the better the flavor and the more nutrients the food contains.

Emphasizing fresh foods also guarantees that you will focus on whole foods, as close as possible to their natural state. Prepackaged flour that has been sitting on a warehouse shelf or in the grocery store for more than a year does not qualify as "fresh" food, nor does a box of "buffalo-helper" with noodles, artificial flavors, and preservatives. In most grocery stores, fresh foods line the outer walls while packaged foods fill the middle aisles. Spend the majority of your time (and your money) in the perimeter of the grocery store. Better yet, plant a garden, even a small one, and cultivate a grocery store in your backyard.

What this means for you:

The fresher the food, the better the flavor and the greater the nutritional value.

SECRET #12:
Cook foods to maximize nutrient absorption.

From Chinese perspective, the stomach is a "warm" organ that "cooks" our food. In order to maximize the stomach's cooking activity, the Chinese suggest eating warm, cooked foods. The foods do not need to be cooked to death, but rather steamed, baked, or stir-fried to gently cook the food. Lightly cooking food, especially vegetables and other fibrous foods, makes them easier to digest and assimilate.

Excessively cold or fatty foods "dampen" the stomach's fire. "Cold" foods include ice water, ice cream, and lots of raw vegetables. Fatty foods such as butter, pork, heavy sauces, and gravies also compromise the stomach's cooking fire. That's why the suggested meal for "how to have indigestion in one easy meal" includes lots of fat and tops off the meal with a frozen dessert.

Raw foods "dampen" the digestive system

You may be surprised that the list of foods that increase dampness includes raw vegetables. Many contemporary diets recommend increasing raw foods, with good reason. Raw foods contain lots of vitamins, minerals, and enzymes. Cooking, especially over-cooking, can destroy some of the nutrients and all of the enzymes. Raw vegetables, however, can be very difficult to digest. Plant cell walls contain cellulose, an indigestible starch. In order to get the full nutritional benefits, you have to break down the cell walls. Most people do not chew raw vegetables well enough to break down the cell walls. They may benefit from the increased fiber but miss the nutrients still trapped inside the plant cells. As mentioned earlier, juicers that use the whole fruit or vegetable can increase nutrient absorption from raw foods without sacrificing the fiber content.

I would suggest eating raw foods according to the cycles of the seasons. In the summer, when the weather is warmer, our bodies can "cook" more raw foods in the stomach. As the weather chills, however, the digestive system has a harder time digesting and assimilating raw foods. Similarly, people who live in warm climates usually can eat more raw foods than those who live in cold, dark, damp climates. Portland, Oregon would not be a good place to start a raw food renaissance. San Diego, California, however, might be an excellent spot for raw food enthusiasts.

Another measure for how much raw food is optimal for you is to watch your body's response. After eating raw foods, watch for signs of "dampness": bloating, loose stools, a heavy feeling in the abdomen, or feeling full after only a few bites of food. As an example, if you eat a large salad with lots of raw vegetables and then have a bloated abdomen and loose stools, you are eating too much raw food.

What this means for you:

Eat small amounts of raw foods during the warm months of the year.

Avoid raw foods during the damp, cold seasons.

Journey to Health

Return to your Journey to Health on page 108 and review your final destination. Consider these questions:

- Has my vision of health changed? Do I want to alter or add anything to my vision?
- How does diet fit into my vision of health?
- What are some of the dietary choices I can make that will support my health?
- Do I have a health care provider trained in nutrition, who focuses on food as well as supplements?
- What dietary changes will support me in creating lifelong health?

Remember that the first step in creating anything in your life is to have a clear vision of what you want. In the "Destination" part of the map, describe your optimal diet.

Diet Diary

After clarifying what you want, the next step is to describe accurately where you are right now. The process of recording what you eat for an entire week can be an enlightening process, helping you create a very clear picture of your diet. During this week, eat as you normally would. Choose a week that is as close to "normal" as possible. A vacation in Hawaii complete with nightly luaus may not be the best week to record your typical diet. A business trip also may not be the best time unless you spend the majority of your time on the road.

Be as astute an observer as you can this week. Record everything that goes into your mouth, including gum, maraschino cherries, and breath mints. Include what you drink as well.

At the end of the week, the diet diary will serve as the starting point, defining "where you are" right now. As you review the diet diary, evaluate the following areas:

- Am I drinking 64 ounces of water a day?
- How many caffeinated beverages am I drinking each day?
- Did I have a positive water balance at the end of the day (two cups of water for every cup of caffeinated beverage *plus* 64 ounces of water)?
- How much animal protein am I eating per day?
- How much plant protein am I eating per day?
- How many saturated fats am I eating (animal and hydrogenated fats)?
- Approximately what percentage of my calories comes from fat? [This may take some calculation. Remember that one gram of fat delivers nine calories, so multiply the number of grams of fat by nine. Divide the number of fat calories (smaller number) by the number of total calories (larger number) to get the percentage of calories that came from fat.]
- How many sweets do I eat on average?
- How often do I eat fast food, and what kind?
- How often do I eat in restaurants?
- What pre-packaged foods did I eat this week (from a vending machine or from the grocery store)?
- On average how many servings of fruits and vegeta-

bles do I eat each day?

- How many servings of whole grains do I eat per day?
- How did I get calcium and other minerals in my diet (e.g. dairy or leafy green vegetables)?
- How much alcohol do I consume on average each day?
- How many cigarettes do I smoke per day?
- What over-the-counter drugs do I take? How much?
- What street drugs do I take? How much?
- What prescription medications do I take? What are they for?

Action Steps

Now that you have a well-defined destination for your diet and a clear view of your current situation, you can make a list of action steps. As you write each step, ask yourself if that step will move you toward your vision of health. Below are a few examples of steps you may choose to take. This is by no means an exhaustive list, just some ideas to stimulate your own creative process. Remember that your path to lifelong health is unique to you and your body.

- Eat one new vegetable or fruit each week for eight weeks.
- Cook one new whole grain dish every week for a month.
- Drink 64 ounces of filtered water per day.
- Eat animal protein three times a week.
- Buy only organic foods.

- Carry healthy snacks in the car for "emergencies."
- Sit down for one meal a day (or every meal).
- Eat beans for breakfast four mornings a week.
- Chew each bite of food 25 times.

Each action step is defined clearly and easy to measure. Having a clear standard by which to measure means you can easily track your progress. "Eat more vegetables," for example, is a vague action. Does "more" mean a carrot stick or a bushel?

Moving On

Because the digestive system is the very core of the body, the interface through which you receive nourishment and discard wastes, these first steps on the journey to your destination are powerful, life-enhancing steps. With optimal nourishment, your body can begin to walk, then skip, and then dance along the path to health. Which brings us to . . .

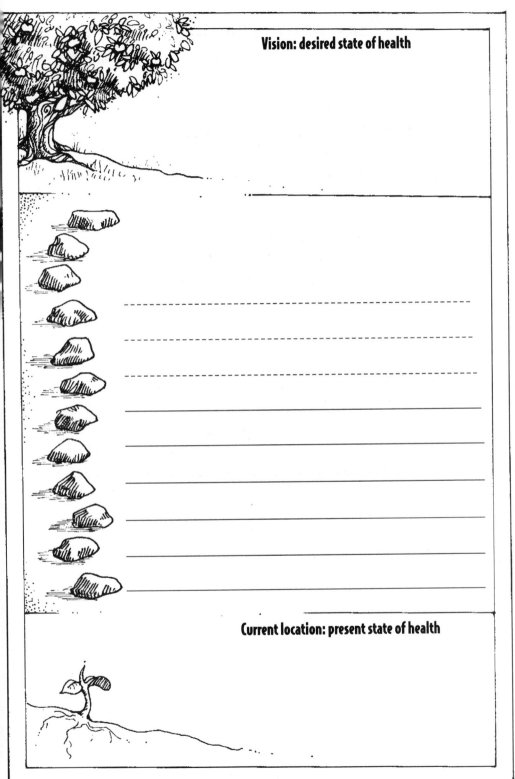

Vision: desired state of health

Current location: present state of health

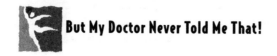 **But My Doctor Never Told Me That!**

NOTES:

CHAPTER 5

Classified Information About Exercise

One afternoon I took a call from a woman potentially interested in joining the High Level Wellness Program©. "What will we be doing in the class?" she asked in her melodious Indian accent.

"The first section of the course focuses on wellness and your vision for health . . ."

"Yes, yes," she said. I could imagine her nodding her head at the other end of the line.

"The second section addresses nutrition . . ."

"Oh, I already know all about that," she said emphatically.

"During the third section we focus on exercise . . ."

"Oh," she said disdainfully, "I am not going to exercise. Thank you very much." She hung up the phone.

This woman's response is fairly typical. Despite the "exercise craze" of the past decade, fewer than 20 percent of the American population exercises regularly. The nomadic peoples of China's northwestern province traditionally spent most of their waking lives on horseback. In the United States, our "horse" is a car, and our favored position is sitting – on a chair, in a car, or on a sofa. Our lives career at magnificent speeds as we chase children, work obligations, and family demands. Amidst all of the activity, however, our bodies remain remarkably still.

Our bodies are made to move. The body rewards even small increments of exercise with a vast array of positive physiological changes.

**SECRET #1:
Exercise effects more than muscles.**

Exercise certainly does strengthen and tone muscles. Physical movement also affects several other body systems including the cardiovascular, digestive, immune, and endocrine systems.

Cardiovascular health and exercise

Thanks to Dr. Kenneth Cooper, who coined the term "aerobics," most people understand how exercise benefits the heart, lungs, and circulatory system. Aerobic exercise, defined more completely below, is any exercise that is rhythmic, utilizes the large muscle groups, and increases heart and breathing rates. Gradually increasing aerobic exercise over time causes the heart and lungs to work more efficiently. The heart pumps more blood with fewer contractions, thereby reducing strain on the heart. Recent research on menopausal women with mildly to moderately elevated blood pressure showed that even moderate aerobic exercise significantly reduced blood pressure. The women walked at a moderate pace for 40 to 45 minutes a day for twelve weeks. Although they did not significantly improve lung capacity,

What this means for you:

Even moderate exercise can have a dramatically positive effect on cardiovascular health.

these women had markedly lower resting blood pressure readings.[1]

SECRET #2:
Exercise boosts the immune system.

Did you know that a daily walk strengthens your immune system as well as your heart? Moderate exercise increases white blood cell activity, particularly the neutrophils.[2,3] Excessive training, however, can reduce neutrophil activity and may decrease resistance to infections.[4] Natural killer cells, important defense cells also linked with cancer prevention, increase after moderate exercise sessions.

Just as we discussed in Chapter 4 about nutrients, our body has a normal "physiological window" for exercise. Too little exercise will not stimulate immune cells, yet too much exercise may deplete the immune system. Like Goldilocks, you are searching for the amount of exercise that is "just right" for your particular body. The "physiological window," that "just right" amount of exercise, will increase the health of your immune system.

What this means for you:

Moderate exercise stimulates the immune system while excessive exercise weakens immune response. More is not always better!

> **SECRET #3:**
> **Exercise improves digestion and**
> **reduces constipation.**

In Chapter 4 we followed food through the entire digestive tract. "Peristalsis," wave-like muscle contractions, move food all the way through the digestive system. Without this wave-like motion, food would stagnate and putrefy in the digestive tract. Exercise increases peristalsis, promoting normal digestion and elimination. For constipation, a daily walk or other regular exercise can promote normal bowel movements.

> **SECRET #4:**
> **Exercise stabilizes blood sugar levels and**
> **can even treat non-insulin dependent**
> **diabetes (NIDDM).**

The endocrine system is made up of all of the glands in the body, including the pancreas, which secretes insulin to normalize blood sugar levels. We discussed earlier how processed "white" foods enter the blood stream like lightening, causing blood sugar to skyrocket and then crash. In those suffering with non-insulin dependent diabetes, insulin receptor sites become resistant to insulin. Receptor sites are like baseball gloves that catch a specific substance. Once bonded with the baseball glove, the substance catalyzes certain activities in the cell. "Resistant" receptor sites do not allow the substance to bond. In essence, the catcher's mitt is closed. When insulin bonds with an insulin receptor site, it acts like a "key," opening the "lock" or cell wall so that blood sugar can enter. Diabetics have high levels of sugar in the blood, but the glucose in the blood cannot penetrate the cells until insulin unlocks the cell wall to allow glucose to enter. Exercise opens the "catcher's mitt" so insulin can bond.

Exercise also stabilizes blood sugar levels by effecting the Basal Metabolic Rate (BMR), the speed at which our bodies "burn" energy. After exercising the BMR remains elevated for up to six hours, which means our bodies burn more calories during that time.

What this means for you:

Exercise stabilizes blood sugar levels and increases the metabolic rate for several hours.

Muscles and bones and exercise (oh my!)

Every time a muscle contracts, the muscle pulls against a bone. This pulling action slightly traumatizes the bone. Osteoblasts, the building cells in the bone, repair these damaged areas and in the process actually strengthen the bone. Without exercise, the bones never get the message to rebuild. Over time, bones lose minerals and decrease in strength. Many menopausal women, concerned about bone health, take lots of calcium and magnesium supplements. Without exercise, however, the bones never get the message to pack those minerals into the bone.

Between ages 35 and 40, women's bones reach peak bone mineral density. The best time to prevent osteoporosis (loss of bone mineral) is in our teens and

What this means for you:

Exercise builds strong bones.

The higher your peak bone mineral density (ages 35 to 40), the better your bone health in later years.

twenties because exercise during our early years increases bone mineral density and helps maximize our mid-life peak. Recent studies demonstrate that a seven to eight percent increase in bone mineral density at our peak (ages 35 to 40), and maintaining that increase through continued exercise, reduces our risk of hip fracture by five times![5] In other words, a lower peak bone mineral density increases risk of fracture in later years, while an increase in peak bone mineral density reduces the risk of fracture. Once we have reached peak bone mineral density, we can help protect bone strength by continuing to exercise regularly. For post-menopausal women, any type of exercise benefits the bones, but the largest increases in bone mineral density are among women who are very physically active.[6] Low to medium physical activity helps maintain but does not significantly increase bone mineral density.

Strong muscles support strong bones. One study found that increased physical activity improved the strength of back muscles and enhanced bone mineral density.[7] Increasing muscle strength, however, is only one aspect of a total exercise program.

SECRET #5:
We need several types of exercise.

Not only is the body made to move, it actually craves (and needs) several different types of exercise.

A complete program includes endurance, strength building, flexibility, and agility or coordination exercises. In the next section we will explore these different types of exercise and relate them to your own personal exercise program.

Endurance exercise:

Endurance measures the body's ability to exercise for an extended period of time. The best endurance building exercise is aerobic activity. Any rhythmic activity that increases heart rate, deepens breathing, and uses the large muscles of the leg qualifies as aerobic exercise. Sudden stop-start activities, such as tennis or volleyball, do not qualify as "aerobic" because they do not maintain the steady, rhythmic pace of aerobic exercises such as walking, swimming, and running.

The "FIT" (Frequency, Intensity, Time) concept outlines the minimum amount of exercise you need to maintain aerobic fitness. If you want to improve cardiovascular fitness, you need to increase these parameters gradually over time:

Frequency: in order to develop cardiovascular fitness, you need to exercise aerobically at least three times a week.

Intensity: refers to how intensely you are working the heart. For beginners the "target heart rate," or recommended intensity, is 60 to 70 percent of maximum heart rate (see below for how to calculate your maximum and target heart rates).

What this means for you:

To maintain basic cardiovascular fitness, follow the F*I*T* concept: exercise aerobically *three times a week *at your target heart rate *for 15 to 20 minutes.

<u>*Time*</u>: your aerobic workout should last at least 15 to 20 minutes. Fitness experts used to think the aerobic activity had to be continuous. Now we are learning that aerobic exercise scattered throughout the day has as much benefit as one concentrated aerobic session. The combination of a ten minute walk with the dog before work, five minutes of climbing stairs during lunch, and another walk with the dog when you get home still qualifies as 20 minutes of aerobic exercise.[8]

<u>*(Length)*</u>: You need to exercise regularly for at least six weeks before you can measure physiological improvements (e.g. increased heart and lung efficiency). Of course, you don't have to wait six weeks to notice lots of other improvements such as deeper sleep, brighter moods, and increased agility.

Maximum and Target Heart Rates

The **maximum heart rate** marks the maximum number of beats per minute your heart can safely endure. Pushing beyond the maximum heart rate may damage your heart. To figure your maximum heart rate, subtract your age from 220:

220 – _____ (your age) = _____ beats per minute (maximum heart rate)

Example of maximum heart rate: Richard is 37 years old. **His maximum heart rate is 220 – 37 = 183 beats per minute.**

At your **target heart rate,** you should still be able to talk while exercising. When exercising at your target heart rate, you receive all the benefits of exercise without straining the heart. For beginning exercisers, the target heart rate is 65 percent of your maximum heart rate.

The **resting heart rate** is the number of times your heart beats in one minute when you are relaxed. You can count your pulse easily at the neck – place your forefinger flat against your neck with the tip pointed upward toward your chin. Slide your finger to the side, into the trough on either side of your throat, and you will easily feel your pulse. Rest your finger lightly against your neck – you don't need to press hard to feel the pulse.

[(220 – your age _____) – resting heart rate _____]
x **.65** + resting heart rate _____ = target heart rate.

Example of target heart rate: Richard is 37 years old. His maximum heart rate is 183 and his resting heart rate is 65 beats per minute.
Target heart rate: [(220-37) – 65] x .65 + 65 = 141.7, or round up to **142 beats per minute.**

For advanced exercisers and athletes, aim for 75 to 85 percent of your maximum heart rate. Use the above formula, but multiply by .75 or .85 instead of .65.

Characteristics of aerobic exercise:
- Rhythmic and continuous
- Uses the large muscles of the body (legs)
- Increases heart rate to target heart rate
- Deepens breathing

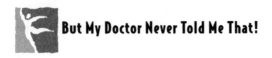

Types of aerobic exercise:

Walking	Bicycling
Jogging or running	Rowing
Swimming	Backpacking
Hiking	Stair climbing

Non-aerobic exercise:

Tennis	Weight lifting
Basketball	Water-skiing
Volleyball	Wind surfing
Baseball	Horseback riding
	(the horse gets the aerobic points!)

These non-aerobic exercises develop other important aspects, e.g. eye-hand coordination or strength, but they do not qualify as aerobic exercise.

Strength-building exercise

Strength-building exercise increases the muscles' ability to exert force against resistance, e.g. lifting an object or throwing a ball. Over time, strength building exercise increases muscle size. Because men have higher testosterone levels, they develop larger muscles more quickly. Women, in contrast, increase muscle strength by 44 percent before their muscles increase in size. For women, strong muscles do not necessarily mean large muscles.

When asked the single most important factor to

slow aging in the body, researcher William Evans immediately responded, "Lift weights." Each year after age 35 our bodies gain 1.5 pounds of fat and lose 0.5 pounds of muscle. Our scales measure the increase in fat but cannot detect the loss of muscle, which affects both our body shape and our metabolism.

At rest, one pound of fat burns approximately two calories a day. In comparison, a pound of muscle burns 34 calories a day! Losing muscle and gaining fat means that our bodies burn fewer calories per day. As our metabolism slows, we convert more of our food calories into fat. We enter a vicious cycle – more fat means fewer calories burned means more food calories converted into fat . . . no wonder we have more trouble maintaining a normal weight after age 35!

Strength building exercise can prevent that 0.5 pound per year muscle loss. You are never too old to begin. Even elderly nursing home residents (ages 86-96) significantly benefited from a weight-training program.[9] With gradual training, you can even increase muscle mass over time.

Research in the early 1990s demonstrated that exercise programs combining aerobic and resistance exercise catalyzed three times more fat loss than aerobic exercise alone. Knowing how many more calories muscles burn at rest, you can understand why resistance exercises, e.g. weight lifting, would increase fat loss.[10]

> What this means for you:
>
> *Weight lifting can reverse the effects of aging by building muscle mass and increasing the metabolic rate.*

	Muscle	Fat
Calories burned at rest	34 calories per pound per day	2 calories per pound per day
Amount lost after age 35 (sedentary)	0.5 pounds per year	0
Amount gained after age 35 (sedentary)	0	1.5 pounds per year

How much do you really weigh?

Stepping on a scale provides limited information about the actual composition of the body – how much of the weight comes from bones? How much from muscle or fat? The scale gives the total weight but cannot report the proportion of different tissues that contribute to that weight.

Many people in this culture become slaves to their scales. Women's magazines make fortunes peddling the latest quick weight loss diets. These programs do work. People lose weight . . . for a short time. Usually within a few weeks of stopping the grapefruit-and-marshmallow-only regime, the frustrated dieter tips the scales at an even higher weight than before she started the diet. Unfortunately during these severe regimens the dieter loses more muscle than fat. Crash dieting catapults the body into "survival" mode. The metabolic rate slows to a crawl to protect the body from starvation. In this crisis situation, the body shifts from burning fat to consuming muscle for calories and protein. When the hapless dieter reaches her target weight, she has slowed her body metabolism to that of a hibernating reptile and reduced muscle tissue in her body. When she returns to her normal diet, her slowed metabolism ensures that her body will quickly replace its lost store of fat plus a little buffer, just in case she encounters "hard times" (another diet) in the future. She also may struggle to maintain even this increased weight because she now has less muscle to burn calories.

Testing body fat percentage

Knowing your percentage of body fat provides more useful information than the scale alone. You can have body fat percentage tested by four different methods:

- The **immersion test** requires a swimming pool and measures the amount of water your body displaces in the pool. For an accurate measurement, you must expel all of the air from your lungs and completely immerse yourself under water. The main problem with this test is that most people cannot completely expel all of the air from their lungs. Otherwise, assuming you can imitate the amazing deflating human balloon, this is a very accurate test.

What this means for you:

Increasing your metabolic rate with aerobic and strength building exercise is a better weight loss strategy than focusing on diet alone.

183

- The **caliper test** measures the thickness of fat folds on the underside of the upper arms, abdomen, or back. Although very inexpensive, the caliper provides only a rough estimate of body fat percentage that is not as accurate as the other two tests.

- **Body composition machines** pass extremely low voltage electricity through the body. The more muscle in the body, the more resistance the current meets. The more the fat, the less the resistance. A high-quality body composition machine comes close to matching the immersion test for accuracy. Some manufacturers claim the body composition machines are more accurate than the immersion tests because they do not rely on completely expelling air from the lungs. Generally the body composition tests cost much less than immersion tests.

- **Home scales** that also measure body fat are convenient but, like the caliper test, only give a rough estimate. Save your money for the body composition machine or immersion tests.

What this means for you:

If you are trying to lose weight, repeat the body composition test every four to six weeks to make sure you are losing fat and not muscle.

Flexibility

Stretching exercise increases the suppleness of joints and muscle tissue. Cats and other animals know the secrets of stretching. Watch a cat or dog indulging in a luxurious stretch after a long nap in the sun. Stretching lubricates joints, increases blood flow in the muscles, and improves flexibility. Lack of flexibility can increase muscle soreness and heighten the chance of muscle injury.

In addition to feeling good, stretching encourages proper muscle repair. Stretching reminds muscle tissue of its normal movement pattern so that the muscle fibers repair in the right direction. Without stretching, an injured muscle protects itself by laying down a tangled mass of connective tissue. This scar tissue can disrupt a muscle's normal movement, leading to pain and reduced range of motion.

As with any type of exercise, our bodies have an optimal range for stretching. Both too little and too much stretching can cause muscles and connective tissue to shrink. What is the right amount? Aim for at least five minutes of stretching per day. As we age, stretching becomes an increasingly important part of our exercise routine to keep muscles and joints supple.

In addition to stretching, our bodies need "range-of-motion" (ROM) exercises, meaning activities that take a joint through its full scope of movement. The shoulder, for example, can extend forward, above, and backward; reach to the side; and rotate in a circle. The wrist can flex forward and to the side, extend backward, and rotate. Static holding stretches improve the flexibility of the muscle in the direction stretched. ROM exercises remind muscles of their normal motions and stimulate correct muscle repair. In addition, ROM exercises increase the production of fluids that

What this means for you:

For those recovering from muscle tears or strains, work with a physical therapist who can coach you on the exercises most appropriate for you. Start a therapeutic exercise program ONLY with expert guidance.

lubricate the joints, which helps to maintain the strength and flexibility of the joints. ROM exercises can stimulate the repair of old muscle tears or strains even years after the injury.

Stretching pointers:
- Warm muscles before stretching. Exercise warms muscles by increasing blood flow. Stretch gently before exercising and then stretch more intensively at the end of your exercise session when the muscles are warm. You also can soak in a hot bath, sauna, or take a steam bath to warm muscles before stretching.
- Stretch to the point that you feel you could hold the stretch forever; do not stretch to the point of pain.
- Never bounce when stretching. "Ballistic" stretching may over-stretch a muscle and cause muscle tears.
- Breathe into a stretch. Allow the body to relax and gradually increase the stretch.

Range of motion pointers:
- Move each joint through its full range of motions two or three times a day.
- Move SLOWLY and smoothly.
- When moving the neck, for example, bend forward and then slowly backward. On the backward extension, lift the chin rather than letting the head drop back against the shoulders (this protects the nerves and muscles in the back of the neck). Looking straight ahead, bend the neck to the side, with the ear toward the shoulder. Return to center. Slowly turn, looking over the shoulder, as far as you can

stretch comfortably. Slowly and smoothly rotate the neck rather than jerking and trying to "pop" the neck.

- If you are restricted in moving certain joints, move as fully as you can without pain. Over time, you will be able to move farther and more freely.
- Rather than trying to complete many repetitions, repeat fewer times moving the joint to its maximum comfort range.

Coordination or agility

A fourth major component of an exercise program is the development of neuromuscular coordination, also called "agility." Sports that require eye-hand coordination fine-tune the connection between nerve signals and muscle response. Balancing activities, such as walking across a beam or log, also spur nerve-muscle coordination. Gymnasts refine this exercise proficiency to an art form. Yoga routines usually include at least one balance exercise to develop this skill.

Early in our childhood development, we moved unilaterally – our right hand moved forward with our right leg when we first learned to crawl. Babies reach an important developmental milestone when they begin to "cross-crawl," moving the right arm with the left leg. Moving opposing limbs stimulates a variety of nerve centers in the brain.

Suggestions for coordination exercises:

- Include cross-crawl exercises in your warm up routine before exercising. These exercises prime the brain as well as the body for peak performance. An example of a cross-crawl exercise is lifting the left knee while swinging the right arm forward. Next lift the right knee and swing the left arm forward. Repeat six to ten times.

- Practice balancing for at least a couple of minutes a day. Alternately stand on one leg and then the other at the bus stop. Follow a crack in the sidewalk like a tight rope walker. Set up a low beam in your back yard with a 2 x 4 and a couple of bricks.

- Many children's toys develop eye-hand coordination. Revisit childhood favorites such as yo-yos, paddle boards, jacks, Frisbee™, or hopscotch. If you have kids, join them in these games. The paddleboard provides great stress relief as well as a fun way to develop eye-hand coordination. Keep one in your desk and spend a minute paddling to unwind after a difficult meeting with your boss.

- Any sport that involves catching, kicking, or hitting develops coordination. Examples include tennis and all racquet sports, soccer, baseball, handball, and football.

"I'm not an athlete. I dreaded gym class in school. How can I create an exercise program that works for me?"

The good news is that you don't have to be an athlete to create an enjoyable exercise program. In fact, athletes may not be the best models for developing an exercise program. Because they are focused more on performance than overall health, most athletes spend the majority of their training time on only one or two types of exercise. The tennis pro, for example, may develop strength and coordination but lag in flexibility. The yoga teacher may excel at flexibility and balance exercises but score poorly on cardiovascular fitness. An athlete also requires more training time than those of us who exercise for our health's sake.

A good exercise program includes all four types of exercise (endurance, flexibility, strength building, and coordination) either within one exercise session or over the course of a week.

Endurance: Remember the FIT (Frequency, Intensity, Time) concept. For minimum cardiovascular fitness, exercise aerobically three times a week for 15 to 20 minutes at your target heart rate.
Stretch: for at least five minutes a day.
Strength building: include strength building exercise two to three times a week.
Agility: include at least two minutes of coordination or balancing exercise each day, which could be flipping a

Frisbee™ with the kids or doing a balancing yoga posture such as The Tree.

TOTAL TIME PER WEEK (to maintain basic fitness): 170 minutes. That translates to an average of 25 minutes a day – less time than you spend watching your favorite news program or sit-com!

If you use the videos suggested in Appendix B, you will combine endurance, strength building, and stretching exercise in the same session.

Tips for starting an exercise program

- Choose types of exercise you love. Many patients look genuinely surprised when I suggest the activities they most enjoy could be wonderful sources of exercise. "You mean dancing counts as exercise?" asked one incredulous patient. "Of course," I told her, "as long as you are moving steadily, increasing your heart rate, and breathing deeply. You can even dance in your own living room – you don't have to go to a dance studio."
- Incorporate exercise into your daily life. The more easily you can include exercise in your daily life, the more likely you will be to maintain a regular program. You don't have to squeeze into Lycra tights and drive across town to a gym to exercise. Of course if you enjoy exercise clubs, by all means join a club. If you live far away from an exercise gym or don't like the atmosphere, you can discover many other ways to

include exercise in your daily routine. If you live in town, consider walking to the post office or grocery store instead of driving. Walk the dog twice a day instead of once; perhaps over time the pace can increase to a jog or a run. Work in the garden. Rake leaves. Shovel snow – one of the most challenging strength building, aerobic exercises around! Play your favorite music and dance in the living room, with or without your sweetie. Check out exercise videos at the public library (see Appendix B for recommendations). Because of time and money constraints, I abandoned my health club membership in favor of a series of extremely effective exercise videos that I can do any time I please, in my own home.

- Begin slowly! Many people in their zeal to begin a new program push themselves too far the first day or week of a new exercise program. The first day the body seems remarkably fit. You may easily surpass your initial goals. Twenty-four to 48 hours after that first walk or weight lifting session, however, you may vow never to don your sweats again. At that point, sore muscles and aching joints may be painful reminders of your over-exertion.

- I really do mean "slowly." Someone who has not exercised for years, for example, might begin with a five-minute walk every day. The second week he could increase to a seven-minute walk, the third week to eight or nine minutes a day. Better to begin with small, attainable goals and gradually increase activity than experience the agony of running three miles the first day out. Weekend warriors may only exercise on weekends because they are too sore to do more than crawl to work during the week. In addition, suddenly exerting the body increases the likelihood of damaging a joint, tearing a muscle, or overtaxing the heart.

- If you cannot find a continuous block of time to exercise, break up your exercise program into smaller time segments. An example for the Wonder Woman Working Mom:
  - Walk the dog for five minutes in the morning, followed by five minutes of yoga stretches (e.g. Salute to the Sun). If you don't have a dog, take a short walk anyhow (or borrow the neighbor's dog).
  - Park as far away from the office building as possible and walk across the parking lot.
  - Use stairs instead of the elevator.
  - Spend five minutes climbing stairs during lunch OR take a five-minute walk.
  - In the afternoon, instead of a five-minute coffee break, climb the stairs again.
  - In the evening lift light dumb-bells while watching TV. Encourage your kids to join you.
- For those able to exercise for an extended period, warm up for at least five minutes at the beginning of an exercise session. Stretch gently OR simply begin whatever exercise you are doing at a slower pace. Begin walking slowly for five minutes, for example, then step up the pace to reach your target

heart rate. Warming the muscles reduces later muscle soreness and decreases the likelihood of muscle tears.

- Slow your pace at the end of each exercise session. This slow down period allows your heartbeat and breathing to return to normal. Suddenly stopping exercise may cause blood to pool in the legs and lead to fainting. Continue exercising – just reduce your speed.

- If you are sore, gentle exercise relieves muscle pain more effectively than analgesics (e.g. aspirin). Take a short walk and do a series of gentle stretching exercises. Immediate muscle soreness probably is caused by increased acidity (lactic acid) and prostaglandin production. Delayed onset muscle soreness (24 to 48 hours after exercising) probably is caused by micro-tears in the muscle and connective tissue. Stretching reminds the muscle tissue of its normal function so that the muscle fibers repair in the right direction. Muscles repaired without gentle stretching are more likely to form a mass of criss-crossing fibers, or "scar" tissue, that does not function normally.

- Always do less than you think you can, particularly in the first month of an exercise program. Give your body time to adjust to new activities. Remember you are making changes for a lifetime. If you need an extra month to reach your weight lifting target, who's counting? You will be enjoying the benefits of your exercise program for decades to come, not just in the coming weeks and months.

- Vary the type of exercise. I suggest choosing at least three different types of exercise you enjoy and rotating among them at regular intervals. Exercise studies have demonstrated that aerobic training is specific to the muscle groups exercised. In other words, running five miles a day develops aerobic capacity, but if you suddenly switch to bicycle riding, you will not have as great an aerobic capacity on the bike as you did running. Your body increases aerobic capacity in conjunction with the specific muscles you are training. This research spawned "cross-training" programs to develop multiple muscle groups and enhance aerobic capacity.

Reviewing your Journey to Health

Return once again to your Journey to Health chart.
1. Review your destination.
   - Has my vision of health changed?
   - Do I have more insight into how I want to look and feel?
   - If I could inhabit this vision, would I choose it?
   - Do I need to add or subtract anything from my health destination?
2. Take stock of your current location.
   - How has my diet changed?
   - Has my digestion improved?
   - On a scale of one to ten, how would I rate my overall energy (with ten representing my full, vibrant energy)?

- Re-examine the exercise journal from the beginning of the program.
- What are my favorite types of exercise?
- What kinds of activities do I still want to be doing when I'm 85?
- What kinds of activities do I need to do now so that I can still do everything I want to at 85?

3. Create a picture of optimal health. Create a picture of your current location. Hold both pictures at once, and notice the difference between where you are and where you want to be.

4. Create action steps that will move you from your current location to your health destination.

- Embrace your favorite types of movement.
- Include aerobic, strength building, stretching, and coordination exercises in your program.
- START SLOWLY.
- Have FUN. Yes, Jello™ wrestling counts as strength-building exercise.

Moving forward

You've tackled some of the most difficult terrain – improving your diet and reacquainting yourself with muscles that may have been MIA since you left high school (or even junior high school if you cleverly substituted study hall for gym). By now you may have noticed some significant improvements in your energy, mood, and sleep. Having championed the physical territory, we turn now to the realm of the intangibles, which can be equally important on this journey to health.

Vision: desired state of health

Current location: present state of health

CHAPTER 6

Secrets Your Doctor Never Told You About Mental and Emotional Health

At one time I was certain that all disease had a spiritual or emotional cause. Over time, however, my certainty has softened into a baffled respect for the mystery of health and disease. I no longer have bold explanations for the cause of all illness or a universal diagnosis for our personal and collective maladies. Lacking good measuring devices for this territory of the mind, heart, and soul, I offer information that has served as a divining rod for my own explorations.

Leave the Pops on the radio

Pop psychology has a prolific band of writers and an avid group of followers who learn to dance with anger, run with wolves, tolerate their alien mate (from Venus or Mars), nurture their inner child, and conquer their addictions. Do people take their inner child to day care, I wonder? Do they claim him or her as a tax deduction? Where do they leave their subconscious during the day? Under the pillow? Has anyone proven that the subconscious and unconscious exist? We swallow a lot of pop psychology on faith, hoping for a quick and certain cure for our emotional discomforts. Always the carrot dangled before us is the promise of happiness, satisfaction, peace, and serenity.

A host of pop psychology and pop spirituality books promise nirvana for those of us who

- find and fulfill their purpose
- ask for their desires
- have no desires
- forgive everyone and themselves
- have no expectations of others
  (then what is there to forgive?)
- nurture their inner child
- grow up and "take responsibility" for their lives
- are poor
- are rich
- have lots of great sex (Wilhelm Reich)
- never have sex (Christian saints)
- do what they are "guided" by spirit to do
- do what they want to do
- do what others want them to do
- "get in touch" with themselves
- ignore themselves
- forget themselves

Phew! Yes, I know this is a contradictory list. So which doctrine is correct? Which flavor do you prefer this month? Which one will deliver heaven on earth? Which one will make me happy?

> **SECRET #1:**
> **Focusing solely on emotional responses**
> **impedes the creative process.**

Who says we are supposed to be happy all of the time?

This simple question is a landmine in the world of pop psychology. "But of course we are supposed to be happy," you may think to yourself. "Why else bother with life?"

Happiness, or any other emotion for that matter, is a very slippery measuring stick for life. Emotions are like cloudscapes on a windy day – they come and go, re-form and dissipate, sometimes at a dizzying rate. Arranging life according to emotions guarantees an exciting ride and a revolving-door approach to decision-making. As soon as the clouds shift, so does the decision. How could anyone build a stable life on such an ephemeral foundation?

Robert Fritz, in his book *Creating*, notes, "When people pursue a life dedicated to feeling good, they become overly sensitive to their feelings and can begin to obsess about any changes in their emotions. When they attempt to organize their lives around feeling good or, at least, feeling good about themselves, they prevent true involvement because they are continually analyzing and interpreting their slightest emotional changes, attributing their feelings as belonging to the inner person, the whole person, the feeling person. They then can become paralyzed, limited, narrow, and confused – all because they fear unwanted emotions." [1]

I do not by any means intend to overlook the importance of emotions. Our feelings are powerful forces that color our experience of the world. As we will discuss below, emotions affect our physical bodies. Feelings are an important aspect of the terrain of our lives. Emotions, however, are not the substance of our lives. I am not my emotions; I have emotions. For those dedicated to "exploring" and "healing" emotionally, consider the focus of your lives – on yourself. The focus is not on what you want to create.

Creating what matters is very difficult when you focus on yourself rather than on the object of creation. How can you evaluate the effectiveness of your actions in support of a creation if you are obsessively watching your own reactions? I am not advocating that you ignore emotions, but rather that you view them as part of the landscape, part of the whole of your life. Rather than "How do I feel about that?" perhaps the more important questions are, "What do I want to create? Do I want to create health? Are my actions organized to support health?"

What this means for you:

Emotions color the landscape of our lives. Constantly changing, emotions are poor measures for the effectiveness of our actions.

"If I'm focused on creating something, won't my life get easier?"

In the last month I have had to apply Secret #1 in my own creative process. For two-and-a-half years I have been working on the creation of a series of wellness centers. During the past year I have lost a close family member, contracted Lyme disease, made a major career change, endured bitter disappointments in personal relationships, and survived a major car wreck. In November I began to despair, sinking into a deep depression. "If I'm doing the right thing," I said to myself, "focusing on what I want to create, why are so many horrible things happening in my life?" I began to doubt my decisions and wondered if I was meant to be doing something else. "Is the Universe trying to tell me to give up on this project?" I asked myself. Surely if I were doing "the right thing," life would corroborate, supporting me in bringing this creation to fruition.

I had to remind myself that my emotional state is not a good barometer for the validity of my vision. My emotional roller coaster is an even less appropriate measure for my progress in realizing the vision. This creation requires me to trek through new territory and become a humble student again. I have to acquire and practice skills that are foreign to me. A career counselor would probably advise me to reapply what I already know, using the talents I have already honed to best advantage. Sticking with what I know, however, ensures that I will remain within the boundaries of my current skills, never realizing the visions that are most important to me.

On this journey to health, some days we may feel happy and other days deeply depressed. Euphoria, anxiety, dissatisfaction, anger, and happiness may arise and fade within a week, or even within a few hours. When we evaluate our progress in creating health according to our emotional responses, we are standing on shaky ground.

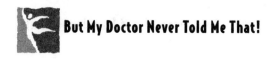
Creating is not therapy

Robert Fritz suggests that ". . . creating is not therapy, not psychology, not New Age philosophy, not religion, not a science, and not a method to bring you riches, happiness, rewards, and success. It is a method for you to bring creations into the world. Creating is not designed to heal you, fix you, or satisfy you, but a way in which you can bring your talents, energies, actions, imagination, reason, intuition, and, yes, even love to the creation you desire."[2]

Perhaps the most important questions for those seeking health are:

- Do I love this vision of health enough to organize my life around creating health?
- Am I interested in creating health for the sake of health?
- Do I want to be healthy in order to support my other life aspirations?
- Am I creating health for me, or am I hoping for rewards in other areas of my life, e.g. the approval of friends, family, or colleagues?

Choosing to be healthy improves your chances of creating health. The choice, however, does not guarantee that the journey will be easy or even that you will reach the final destination. You will not know for sure if you can fulfill your vision of health until you arrive. Choosing health sets the compass and improves your chances of reaching your desired destination.

What this means for you:

Choosing to be healthy and taking action increases the likelihood that you will be healthy.

A choice, however, does not guarantee that you will achieve your goal.

> **SECRET #2:**
> **Exercise and nutrition reduce mental and emotional stress.**

I carefully ordered the chapters in the book to support your overall health. Often improving diet and increasing exercise will eliminate many of the symptoms of chronic stress. Diet and exercise do not eliminate stress but rather increase the body's capacity to tolerate stress. A healthy diet and sound exercise program increase the "ballast" in our lives. This chapter is the "clean up crew," offering ways of addressing the stress that remains even after improving overall health with diet and exercise.

Psychodietetics, published in the 1970s, was the first popular book to link our emotional state with our diet. The author provides countless examples of extreme emotional imbalances treated with simple nutritional changes.

In the 1980s *Sugar Blues* alerted us to the mood-altering effects of simple sugars. The sudden spikes in blood sugar followed by the inevitable blood sugar crashes produce a whole series of physiological and emotional changes in the body. Anyone who has experienced hypoglycemia (low blood sugar resulting from the overproduction of insulin), or who has lived with someone suffering with hypoglycemia, can attest to the debilitating mood swings that accompany the extreme rise and fall of blood sugar levels.

In Chapter 4 we discussed the effects of the two nervous systems in the body, the "Generalissimo" sympathetic nervous system and the "Spa Queen" parasympathetic nervous system. Remember that any kind of stressful situation triggers the Generalissimo, whether the stress is physical or emotional. If you are not used to a cold climate and spend an entire day on the ski slopes, the Generalissimo will kick into gear, commanding increases in norepinephrine [nor-ep-i-NEF-rin] (a.k.a. "adrenalin") and other stress-related hormones so that the body can endure the new, stressful circumstances. Generalissimo also orders blood to flow away from the internal organs and into the muscles, preparing the body to fight or flee from the unwanted circumstances. In this case, as you ski down the mountain you will use the stress-related hormones so that by the end of the day you probably will feel relaxed and happily tired after your day on the slopes.

In contrast, consider the office worker who has just endured an "attack" by an angry boss. Generalissimo does not distinguish physical and emotional stress. From the General's view, a bear in the woods looks remarkably similar to your angry boss. Prepared for the worst, Generalissimo orders the adrenal glands to dump stress-related hormones into the blood stream. The General is preparing for an all-out attack or a quick retreat. Blood quickly flows away from the digestive system and into the muscles. The pupils constrict. Blood pressure rises as blood vessels constrict. You take quick, shallow breaths. The Pad Thai you ate for lunch sits like a rock in your stomach. Your head may throb with increased blood flow.

The best thing for you to do would be to move, to use up the stress-related hormones in physical activity. Office policy, however, dictates that you stay at your desk and continue to be "productive." With sour stomach and throbbing head, you return to the report you were writing. An hour later you have managed to cross out three sentences and write one. You watch the clock, willing the hands to move faster so that you can safely leave the office. "Maybe 4:30 instead of 5 P.M. today?" you bargain with yourself. Once home, you collapse on the sofa and eat a bag of chocolate chip cookies. Still bloated from lunch, the cookies sit like a boulder in your stomach.

A more effective way to work with the stress might be to take a 15 minute "coffee break" and run around the block a few times. If you cannot go outside, run up and down stairs, do sit-ups, push-ups, or any other exercise that space permits. If these incidents happen frequently, keep a jump rope in your desk. Find an empty office or conference room and jump rope for a few minutes. Any physical activity will begin to shift the balance away from Generalissimo's control back toward the realm of the Spa Queen.

Regular daily exercise ensures we do not accumulate a backlog of the stress-related hormones. As an example, a daily walk or other physical activity reduces high blood pressure.[3] Remember that the Generalissimo response

What this means for you:

The more stress you are under, the more important exercise becomes. Exercise uses up the stress-related hormones.

causes blood vessels to constrict, which in turn causes blood pressure to skyrocket. Exercise modulates the stress-related hormones, dilates blood vessels, and helps return blood pressure to normal. Regular exercise tips the see-saw of the sympathetic/parasympathetic nervous systems toward the parasympathetic nervous system. When the Spa Queen holds court, the body sends blood into the internal organs, allowing tissues to repair and regenerate. The Spa Queen demands increased digestive secretions, more nutrient absorption, and efficient waste removal. Her Highness slows the heart rate, dilates blood vessels, and deepens breathing. Under the Queen's reign, the body relaxes and regenerates, increasing its treasure-trove of health.

SECRET #3:
Emotions affect our internal organs, and our internal organs affect our emotions.

Mary, an attractive woman in her late 30s, sat in the reception area reading a book. Her shoulders hunched forward like a protective cape. When I greeted her, Mary gave me a thin smile and then quickly looked at the floor. With her hands stuffed in her jacket, she dutifully followed me down the hall to the treatment room.

We talked about her health and the recurrent bouts of depression that haunted her with increasing frequency. The first episode of depression came in her early twenties. Several years passed before a second episode. Now, in her late thirties, the depression descended on an annual basis, the most recent episode beginning in July, the height of summer sun and heat in Oregon. Because her depression began in the summer, Seasonal Affective Disorder (SAD), a common winter malady in the Pacific Northwest, was an unlikely diagnosis.

After carefully recording all of her physical symptoms, I asked what had been happening in her life in the past year. "Well," she said, "about a year ago I was deciding whether or not to move back in with my husband."

My mind raced back to her earlier mention of gall bladder problems. "Was that a difficult decision to make?" I asked.

"Very," she said, sighing. "I finally decided to move back in with him and our son. I'm going to therapy now, to make sure that I get what I need out of the relationship. That's my responsibility, I know that."

"I'm not surprised that you would be having gall bladder problems during a time like that."

She looked mystified.

"From Chinese medical thinking," I explained, "each internal organ has a positive and negative emotion associated with it. One emotion supports the organ's function, the other undermines it. In Chinese medicine the gall bladder is the 'general,' the one responsible for making decisions. If you doubt yourself, or have a hard time making decisions, you undermine the strength of the gall bladder. The emotion that supports the gall bladder is courage and the ability to make and follow through with decisions."

"Oh," she said, surprised, "that makes a lot of sense. I was having a horrible time making this decision."

"The link between the emotions and the organs is a two-way street," I explained. "The emotion can effect the organ, and the organ can give rise to the emotion. Having a hard time making decisions can weaken the gall bladder, and someone with gall bladder disease may begin to doubt themselves and have a hard time making decisions."

Treating the body through the emotions

Ancient Taoist medical practitioners understood the intimate connection between physical and emotional health. These natural medicine practitioners aimed to treat the root of an illness and knew that in many cases changing an emotional pattern would bring the deepest healing. The Taoists also knew that transforming the mind and emotions could be extremely difficult for patients, so they "entertained" them with acupuncture, herbs, and other physical treatments until patients were ready to change the underlying emotions. The physical treatments could also prepare someone to make the necessary mental or emotional changes.

The Chinese describe our physical processes much more poetically than does western medicine, yet many of the eastern and western explanations share common understandings. From a Chinese medical perspective stress, anger, and depression all affect the liver. Both Western and Chinese medical practitioners observe that

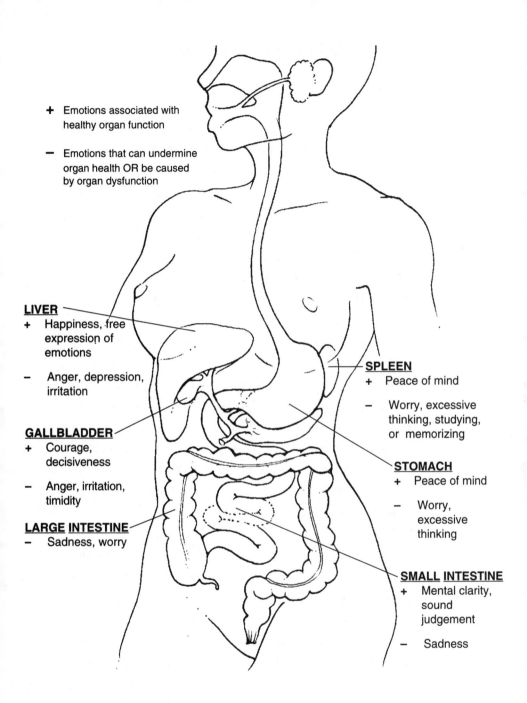

+ Emotions associated with healthy organ function

− Emotions that can undermine organ health OR be caused by organ dysfunction

LIVER
+ Happiness, free expression of emotions

− Anger, depression, irritation

GALLBLADDER
+ Courage, decisiveness

− Anger, irritation, timidity

LARGE INTESTINE
− Sadness, worry

SPLEEN
+ Peace of mind

− Worry, excessive thinking, studying, or memorizing

STOMACH
+ Peace of mind

− Worry, excessive thinking

SMALL INTESTINE
+ Mental clarity, sound judgement

− Sadness

The effects of emotions on the digestive system (Chinese Five Element Theory)

patients with liver problems (e.g. hepatitis, alcoholic cirrhosis, or liver cancer) are often depressed and angry. As the liver degenerates, these emotions become more prevalent. Conversely, someone suffering with anger and/or depression may have reduced liver function as reflected in the more subtle diagnostic methods of Chinese medicine, specifically tongue and pulse diagnosis. Depression usually will not cause changes in the liver that can be recorded with western testing methods, such as blood work. The depressed person, however, may notice more subtle changes, such as sluggish digestion or a vague "ache" just below the ribs on the right where the liver is located. For Mary, we chose to work with acupuncture and certain Chinese herbs to support her liver. Over time we will discover the roots of her depression and the mix of physical, mental, and emotional elements that contribute to her condition.

Digging out the roots of disease

Gardeners know that weeds must be removed entirely, roots and all, or they quickly regrow. Like a weedy garden, we can treat illnesses most effectively by removing the cause, or "root" of the illness. So what is the cause of disease? The answer varies with each individual and each condition. Often multiple factors contribute to the cause.

Contrary to some of the pop spirituality explanations of illness, not all diseases are rooted in mental or emotional patterns. Sometimes we develop a stomach ulcer because we don't rinse our dishes carefully enough (eating traces of the alkaline soap can neutralize helpful stomach acids), not because we hate our job or our mate. Regardless of the cause, illnesses are not "all in the head"– they are connected with our bodies, too. The good news is that the mind-body connection is a multi-way street. Supporting physical health can alleviate emotional distress, and changing emotional patterns can alter our physical health. I don't believe that emotions are the cause of all illnesses any more than I believe physical disorders are the root of all sickness. Health is a combination of physical, mental, emotional, and spiritual health. The challenge is to learn which street, or streets, will lead toward health.

SECRET #4:
Our thoughts, our immune function, and
our nervous system all affect each other.

For generations we have known that thoughts, feelings, and physical health are intimately entwined. Only in the last generation, however, have we had the ability to identify the messengers in the body that link our mind, nervous system, endocrine glands, and immune system. Researchers in this newly emerging science are discovering shape-shifting molecules that communicate between these four major systems in the body. Certain substances in the body, for example, may act as neurotransmitters *and* immune system messengers. We are discovering that the physiological systems in our body are open rather than closed systems. The digestive system influences the endocrine system which in turn affects the nervous system. The links go on and on, weaving one network into another. The body functions much more as a "whole cloth" than the compartmentalized systems approach presented in most physiology textbooks.

As an example, depression has a profound effect on all of our body systems. Researchers following 1,250 depressed patients for up to 19 years discovered that the higher people scored on a depression scale, the higher their risk of dying of heart disease. Those with moderate to severe depression also had an increased risk of dying from any cause compared with those who were not depressed.[4]

The links between the mind, body, and emotions are two-way, or more accurately multi-way streets. The multilingual molecules that communicate between several systems in the body can influence heart disease and depression as well as acute conditions like colds, the flu, and indigestion.

How to catch a cold in only two (exhausting) days

Here is a simple recipe for catching a cold: decide to spend Thanksgiving with your family in Duluth, Minnesota. Board a plane in Seattle, two time zones away, on the busiest travel day of the year. Stand in line with 300 other people, directly behind a woman with two small children who sneeze incessantly. Board the plane and sit next to the man with a barking cough. Watch while he fills the seat pocket with used tissues. Breathe deeply while the plane is taxiing down the runway, inhaling extra carbon monoxide. Buy two wine coolers and doze off during the remainder of the flight.

Arrive in Duluth dehydrated from breathing recirculated air and drinking alcohol. Have a hard time falling asleep (after all, you are now two hours ahead of your usual schedule), and wake up with a stiff back. Make polite conversation with your parents until your brother arrives. Start an argument about who flattened the neighbor's mailbox when you were eight and ten years old. During dinner eat everything in sight while reliving all of your childhood traumas – potatoes boiled in your failure to make the junior high school cheerleading squad, turkey basted in the bitterness of your two-timing 10th grade boyfriend, etc. After dinner sit in misery watching your favorite football team lose in the Banana Bowl.

Go out for a walk as the snow begins to fall. Return home with soggy boots, chilled to the bone. Refuse the extra sweater your mom offers. At dinnertime eat again even though you are not hungry. Play a game of Crazy Eights with the uncle who always sits on some of the cards so no one can win. At 10 P.M. crawl into bed and spend the next two hours tossing and turning before finally falling asleep.

The recipe includes physical "insults" such as dehydration, lack of sleep, and cold exposure. Emotional traumas, such as arguing with a brother and reliving childhood experiences, also play a role. Remember that the digestive system shuts down when we are under stress. The huge holiday meal sours in the digestive tract, producing toxins that affect the rest of the body. The sneezing children and coughing man provide only the seed of illness; the physical and emotional traumas prepare the soil. The bacteria and viruses that cause infections surround us all the time. Only when the immune system is challenged beyond its ability to defend the body does the bacteria or virus gain a foothold and foment an infection.

SECRET #5:
Sleep is your greatest ally in improving
energy and mood.

For years I have been searching for ways to shorten my sleeping hours. Why "waste" time in bed when I could be doing other things? Exercise and meditation advocates claim that these activities reduce the need for sleep. True, exercise increases endorphins and relaxes the body, while meditation induces the alpha and theta brain wave patterns associated with sleep. In the end, though, no activity replaces the rejuvenating benefits of sleep.

James Maas, Ph.D., in his book *Power Sleep* makes a convincing case for devoting more of our precious hours to sleep. According to Dr. Maas, most of us move through our lives like sleepwalkers with decreased mental acuity and alarmingly diminished performance because of our lack of sleep.

When we fall asleep, our brain wave patterns shift from quickly cycling beta waves that characterize wakefulness to progressively slower wave cycles: alpha, theta, and finally delta brain waves. During the third and fourth stages of sleep (theta and delta waves), our body temperature decreases and metabolic activity slows. Growth hormone secretion increases, making these deep stages of sleep particularly important for children and teenagers. Because elders spend less time in deep sleep, they produce less growth hormone. After hard physical activity or sleep deprivation, we spend more time in stage 3 and 4 deep sleep.[5]

Deep sleep also boosts the immune system, particularly the activity of interleukins and tumor necrosis factor (TNF).[6] Even modest sleep loss can reduce the body's immune response[7] and decrease our resistance to viral infections. The less we sleep, the more likely we are to develop a cold or the flu.

During our sleep hours we move from stages 1 (light sleep) through 4 (deep sleep) and then back to stage 1 again, completing this cycle four or five times in a night. During REM (rapid-eye-movement) sleep our body remains motionless while the brain actively dreams. Although dreams can occur at any time during sleep, dreams during REM sleep tend to be more vivid. Several physiological changes in the brain during REM sleep indicate that this stage is vital for memory retention and organization. REM activity increases after periods of intensive learning.[8] Memory retention improves dramatically after a period of REM sleep compared to sleep without REM activity or an equal time awake.[9]

How do I know how much sleep I need?

According to Dr. Maas, most of us need at least eight hours of sleep.

The average adult sleeps between seven and eight hours. For a very few individuals, six hours of sleep each night might be adequate. One or two people in one hundred can manage to get by with five hours. For a significant number of others it might take as many as nine or ten hours of sleep to function at full capacity and be wide awake all day. . . . Realistically speaking, most of us aren't willing to balance our schedules in order to get the optimal ten hours of sleep mentioned in the last chapter. At minimum most people absolutely need to obtain at least sixty to ninety minutes more sleep than they presently get. . . . Dr. Thomas Roth, at Henry Ford Hospital's Sleep Disorders and Research Center in Detroit, found that sleeping one hour longer boosted a person's alertness by 25 percent! And that's just one of the innumerable benefits of getting more sleep.[10]

What this means for you:

To improve memory and alertness, sleep at least one more hour each night.

To discover your sleep quotient, note whether you need an alarm clock to wake up, have a hard time getting out of bed, or feel groggy during the day. If you answer yes to any of these three cues, you need more sleep. When you wake without an alarm clock and feel alert all day, you are getting enough sleep.

Sleep hygiene

Go to bed and get up at the same time every day. Trying to catch up on sleep on the weekends throws off the body clock. After a long slumber on Saturday night, you may have a hard time falling asleep Sunday night. On Monday you awake groggy, short on sleep as you begin the work week.

Reserve your bed for sleep and sex only. If you spend time in bed studying, reading, or eating, your body begins to associate the bedroom with activities other than sleep. Save the bedroom for sleeping and making love only. Move your desk or other office equipment and your dishes to another area of the house.

Take a warm bath before bed. Develop your own "slow down" ritual before bedtime, particularly if you have a hard time falling asleep. Some people continue to work, busily completing activities until a few minutes before going to bed and then wonder why they can't fall asleep. For young children story time or a lullaby can be particularly effective to slow the pace and provide a reassuring transition from the activities of the day to the quiet hours of sleep.

Sleep continuously. Sleep loses some of its restorative properties when interrupted, e.g. by young children or the need to urinate frequently. Often those who have difficulty sleeping will snooze during the day and then have a hard time falling asleep at night. This vicious cycle may prolong sleep deprivation. If you have difficulty sleeping, do your best to avoid naps during the day to promote deeper, longer sleep at night. *Catch up on sleep.* Unfortunately one long night of sleep cannot repay all of our sleep debt. Sleeping longer on the weekends also cannot completely redress sleep deprivation during the week. Most people need five or six weeks of increased sleep to repay completely their sleep debt. For one week move your bedtime to a half an hour earlier while keeping your waking time the same. Increase sleep time by 15 minutes each week until you are fully alert during the entire day. Try reducing sleep by 15 minutes; if you feel sleepy during the day, increase again by 15 minutes.

Once you have repaid your sleep debt, you may have more energy to consider other important aspects of mental/emotional health. Rested and refreshed, you can . . .

SECRET # 6:
Pay Attention to The Big Three.

When asked about the major stresses in their lives, most people name at least one of the following: time, money, and relationships. For more clues about the stressful areas in your personal life, consider completing *The Stress Map* (see information in Appendix B). Each person has a unique pattern of challenges and individualized responses to those stresses. I have chosen the

Big Three based my patients' and my own experience and offer these musings as a catalyst for your own reflections.

"But I don't have enough time!"

Despite the time-saving craze of the 1950s and 1960s, few of us have the luxury of "disposable time." Sadly we are learning that many time-saving devices actually have stolen more time than they have salvaged. The advent of electric vacuums, for example, generated a higher standard of cleanliness for carpets. Homemakers actually spend more time vacuuming with their electrified vacuums than they did with their mechanical carpet sweepers.

When faced with the seductive promises of time-saving devices, calculate whether you really will save time and energy. Will this gadget turn back the clock or simply take up space in a drawer or closet? Can you do the same thing with something you already own? Amy Dacyczyn, author of *The Tightwad Gazette*, had a contest with her husband, testing the speed of microwave versus stovetop popcorn making. Surprisingly, the stovetop method won hands down. High tech does not always guarantee quicker results or greater efficiency.

The paper chase

"I don't have time to read all the stuff that comes in the mail," moans one friend, "much less the newspaper. How am I ever going to keep up with all this information?" I empathize with her. My kitchen table is overflowing with unanswered mail. I have a pile of journals waiting to be read and a two-foot stack of books sitting accusingly next to my desk. No, we have not suddenly become a nation of illiterates, but rather a society overwhelmed with information. One issue of *The Sunday New York Times* contains more information than Benjamin Franklin encountered in his entire lifetime. Franklin was a well-traveled, highly educated man in his day. No wonder we feel overwhelmed with information!

In addition to mastering speed-reading, you can decrease the information glut by focusing on the data that is most important to you. Please don't overlook the wisdom of this simple statement. When you have clear goals for your life and health, you can effectively screen the information cresting in your mailbox, over the radio, or on the TV. Without clear goals, you have no levee for the huge waves of information ready to deluge your time and attention.

What this means for you:

Avoid information overload by focusing on data that serves your goals and discarding the rest.

Open the mail next to the recycling bin, boldly discarding the pieces that do not interest you. If you have a stack of magazines over three months old, discard them. If you have a year's worth of a magazine lying unread, cancel the subscription. Read the first line of each paragraph. Learn to skim information and carefully read only the most important sections.

For those who commute, books on tape offer a way of assimilating information on the go. If you have the choice of purchasing a book or a tape, choose the recorded version.

Finally, if you discard something and then find you need it later, you can almost always resurrect the information.

The Time-Money Game

Most of us spend at least as many hours working as we do sleeping. Executives in fast-paced corporations and stay-at-home moms and dads often work twice as many hours as they sleep. Many of us sacrifice the majority of our waking hours for a paycheck, yet few of us know our true hourly wage.

Vicki Robin and Joe Dominguez, authors of *Your Money Or Your Life*, outline a method for figuring your true hourly wage. Add up ALL of your work-related expenses and subtract them from your paycheck. Include the increased cost of dry cleaning, restaurant meals, convenience foods, childcare, etc. You may be shocked to discover that your real take-home pay may be less than half of your paycheck. After figuring their hourly wages, some couples realize they can save more money with one partner staying at home than they can with both partners working. The stay-at-home partner may "earn" an equal or greater income by cooking meals from scratch instead of depending on restaurant fare, doing laundry, dusting and vacuuming instead of hiring a cleaning service, etc.

Once you know your true hourly wage, you can figure how many "life hours" you pay for an item. Your take-home hourly wage may be $15.00, yet your true hourly wage may be $7.00. When you buy a boom box for $135, you have just spent 19.3 hours of your life!

Joe and Vicki ask fundamental questions about our money and our lives:

- Did I receive fulfillment, satisfaction and value in proportion to life energy spent?
- Is this expenditure of life energy in alignment with my values and life purpose?
- How might this expenditure change if I didn't have to work for a living?[11]

In a consumer-driven society, we rarely ask ourselves these questions. Any advertising agency worth its salt would reply that we never can have enough: "No one can eat just one." Joe and Vicki, however, contend that we can know when enough is enough:

Being fulfilled is having just enough. Think about it. Whether it's food or money or things, if you don't know, from an internal standard, what is enough, then you will pass directly from "not enough" to "too much," with "enough" being like a little whistle-stop town. You blink and you've missed it. You will rarely have an experience of fulfillment. By diligently working with this question you will begin to identify, for yourself, an internal yardstick that you can use to measure how much is enough. . . . **Asking yourself, month in, month out, whether you actually got fulfillment in proportion to life energy spent . . . awakens** that natural sense of knowing when enough is enough.[12]

For those wanting to transform their relationship with money, I highly recommend reading Joe and Vicki's book and following their nine steps to financial independence.

Relationships

Lack of time and money often exacerbate our relationship woes. According to the American Bar Association, 89 percent of all divorces in the United States result from money problems. Having common financial goals can strengthen a partnership and eliminate a host of struggles. If you need a forum for discussing money priorities with your mate, consider creating a "Spending Window" by listing the expenditures you view as "vital," "important," "nice," and "worthless." Compare the lists. You can discover a lot about yourself and your mate simply by creating these windows. You learn what each of you values and how you view money.

Discuss the "vital" and "important" expenditures. If you discover that your number one priority is a new swimming pool while your mate's chief desire is to pay off the mortgage, you may begin to understand why you have conflicts over money. Explore why each of the items is "vital," "important," etc. You may discover that a swimming pool represents more play and fun for you. Perhaps you can incorporate other activities or home improvements that fulfill the same purpose for less money (e.g. a membership at the Y or a basketball hoop in the driveway). Perhaps your mate discovers she wants to pay off the mortgage because she is afraid of future financial problems, e.g. loss of a job or a stock market crash. This revelation gives you an opportunity to discuss security, what you can control in life, and what is beyond your control. Listen respectfully and dig for the root of each item on the "vital" and "important" lists.

What this means for you:

Disagreements about money can bankrupt a relationship. Work together to develop spending priorities.

When you understand what your partner hopes to attain with each item on the list, you can begin to negotiate how best to fulfill those needs and desires. Finally, create a Spending Window with mutually agreed upon "vital," "important," "nice," and "worthless" expenditures. You now have a shared template for making financial decisions.

Time constraints can also burden an otherwise sound partnership. Working partners with children may spend very little time with each other as they coordinate separate work shifts to cover home responsibilities. How can couples maintain their affection and communication with so little contact? Review the information above on figuring your real hourly wage. Do you both truly need to work? Would a stay-at-home mom or dad actually save more money than the additional income would contribute? Of course in some cases both partners absolutely need to work, and they do the best they can to fulfill work and family obligations.

Communities as health insurance

In earlier times the extended family created a "safety net" for struggling families. No one was expected to fend for themselves during times of sickness or other crisis. Without question the community would care for the sick, the wounded, the elderly. In contemporary society, few of us know the unconditional support that many of our ancestors took for granted. For many the binding thread of community has frayed beyond recognition. We have no safety net in times of crisis.

A tightly bonded, caring community is a tremendous health asset. A long-term study on heart disease followed the citizens of Framingham, Massachusetts, to assess the effects of lifestyle on heart disease. Researchers chose Framingham because the residents had an unusually low incidence of heart disease. Careful analysis of diet, exercise, and other lifestyle factors revealed an unexpected factor, the "secret weapon" that differentiated Framingham residents from their neighbors: a strong sense of community support. When Framingham residents moved elsewhere, their risk for heart disease once again rose to the national average. Although they maintained the same diet and exercise program, the absence of a close knit community eroded their health and increased their risk for heart disease.

Ghost Sickness

David Winston, a Cherokee herbalist, speaks of diseases among his people that include sickness of the spirit as well as the body. Those suffering with "Ghost Sickness" have lost contact with Creator, their community, and themselves. Although they still walk among the living, their spirits have atrophied. They may continue to work, yet their bodies are empty shells. One of the chief symptoms is repeating the phrase, "I don't care." Those suffering from Ghost Sickness have lost heart; their spirits are ailing. The Cherokee understand that the spirit is not immortal, but only the individual can kill his or her own spirit. The remedy for Ghost Sickness involves more than pills or herbs. The cure requires a completely new way of living.

Those suffering from Ghost Sickness tend to be self-indulgent, so the medicine person might send them to work in a nursing home or orphanage. The "patient" is encouraged to look at the wider woes of the world. Part of the "cure" is to spend time with disadvantaged people and learn to serve them. The medicine person arranges a series of ceremonies over a period of three or four months to help reconnect the ghost spirit first to family and then to the community. The whole family and then the entire community participate in the ceremonies.

Their presence builds a strong expectation that the person will heal. Many in contemporary Western culture indulge in illness to gain attention. "I'm so sorry you are sick," we say to one another. "What can I do for you?"

Among the Cherokee, friends and neighbors emphasize the healing process. "I'm so glad you are healing," they say. "What can I do for you?"

The Shawnee also share this understanding of emphasizing health. "Always present yourself the way Creator would want to see you," teach the elders. "The way you present yourself is a prayer, a way of thanking Creator for what you have been given. You don't change the body you were given, like piercing holes in it or tattooing it. You honor your body the way Creator made you. Hold a vision of yourself as healthy. See others in health. See them as strong and healthy, because we create with our thoughts." From a Shawnee perspective, you hold a vision of yourself as healthy and take action to fulfill that vision. You thank Creator for the gift of life by caring for your body.

What this means for you:

An ailing spirit needs the "food" of right relationship – with self, family, community, and the larger order of life.

"Birth right" – divinity or delusion?

"You deserve whatever you want," declares a motivational speaker. "In fact, you are entitled to all of the good things you want."

Are we in fact entitled to all that we want? Are we graced with fairy godmothers who effortlessly grant our wishes? Can I have my heart's desire simply by repeating that desire over and over again?

The truth is that we arrive without guarantees or warranties. Our lives are subject to forces we cannot always control. I have yet to find my warranty tag or my money-back guarantee (maybe they came off in my first bath). I have yet to find a universal doctrine that guarantees my entitlement to *anything*.

For the last couple of years I have been struggling with this idea of entitlement. The first sacred cow to fall was the belief that I am entitled to my parents' love. "But wait!" you may scream. "Aren't parents supposed to love their children?" Parents are responsible to care for children, to provide shelter and food and clothing. Love is a side benefit that may or may not come with the package. Some people spend years in therapy reviling their parents' lack of affection. Love is an act of grace, a gift that cannot be commanded. From this perspective, the treasure of love becomes more precious. Rather than an obligation, love becomes an unexpected gift, an offering of divine delight.

Many religious and spiritual doctrines direct us to "love one another," to "love our neighbor as ourselves," and to pray for others but not ourselves in the circle of life. These doctrines tell me that our religious foremothers and forefathers thought we would not naturally love each other. They feared the worst in others' behavior. Otherwise, why would they frame such doctrines? Our religious forebears did not worry about our ability to take care of bodily functions: Thou shalt defecate when you feel an urge. Thou shalt urinate when your bladder is full. Thou shalt eat when you are hungry. No, they did not need to create religious dogma about what they considered to be "natural" functions. The admonitions about loving others, however, tell me that religious leaders of the past did not consider love and concern for others to be a normal, natural part of living. Instead, love became an obligation, a spiritual requirement, a communal burden.

Over time I have dropped the belief that I am entitled to love or the fulfillment of my desires. Rather than expecting certain behaviors from others, I see acts of kindness as fortuitous gifts. I give thanks for those who come to my aid. I rejoice in the manifestation of my goals and visions. I feel gratitude for my family's love. I have nothing to forgive, for forgiveness assumes an unfulfilled obligation from which I am granting amnesty. I can establish structures, take action, and increase the likelihood of achieving my visions. The ultimate fulfillment of those visions, however, is an act of grace, and not a guaranteed outcome.

Freedom

Do you value freedom? What does freedom mean to you? If you value freedom, how do you view other people's choices? Are people free to make choices that differ from your own values? Valuing others' freedom means just that – they are free to do (or not do) as they choose, as long as their actions do not physically harm others. People become people rather than pawns or gratification machines.

What this means for you:

Love is a gift that cannot be commanded. When present, love is an act of grace. No one, not even a parent, "owes" us love.

Freedom also affects relationship with self. What do I really want to do? In the past I believed that having a "vision" automatically implied an obligation to fulfill that inspiration. I am learning that I may have a vision or goal and yet choose not to complete it. I am free to do or not do as I please.

Freedom and health

Review your health goals with freedom in mind. You are free to create health or not. You may have a desire to be healthy but choose not to act on it. Take a moment to tell yourself the truth:

- Do I want to be healthy?
- Do I want to be healthy in order to complete other goals in my life?
- Am I choosing health for its own sake?
- Am I expecting some kind of return on my investment, a reward for improving my health?
- Do I want to take action on my health goals?
- Do I think that I can attain my health goals simply by thinking about them?
- Do I have a clearly defined destination?
- Have I created appropriate measurements to evaluate my progress?
- By when do I want to complete my steps?

Remember you can have a goal and choose NOT to act on it. Simply having an idea or a desire does not necessarily mean you have to fulfill it. You are free to decide whether or not to enact your desires.

Reviewing Your Journey to Health

Health destination
- Revisiting my vision of health, are these goals still important to me?
- Do I need to be healthy in order to fulfill my life goals?
- Revisit your vision of health and ask, "Is this still where I want to go?"
- Have I already completed some of my initial goals?
- How close am I to my vision of health?
- Add or subtract elements as needed.

Current location
- What steps have I taken since I first developed my vision of health?
- How has my body responded?
- What measurements am I using to judge my response?
- How accurately am I measuring my progress?
- Review the exercise journal, diet diary, and exercise questionnaire from Chapter 3.
- What does my diet look like now?
- Has my exercise program changed?
- Complete *The Stress Map* or use some other method to evaluate your current stress levels. See Appendix B for ordering information.

Action Steps to Health
- What steps will I take on my continued journey to health?

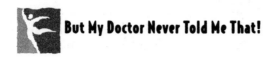

- Are the measurements appropriate to the goal?
- Which steps have been effective so far?
- Which actions have failed to move me forward or diverted me on my journey?
- What steps will move me closer to my vision?

Take a few moments to answer these questions and then modify your Journey to Health as needed.

Vision: desired state of health

Current location: present state of health

Moving on

During this journey you have been exploring the territory of health, delving first into a classical approach to wellness. After familiarizing yourself with the terrain, you created a personal vision for health. You carefully placed stepping stones on the path, evaluating and adjusting as you went. As you move forward, ask yourself, "Why do I want to create health?" Tell yourself the truth about what you want, and decide whether you love the creation enough to devote yourself to its realization. Love and truth are the wellspring that inspires the creative process.

I hope these musings about mental/emotional health will encourage you to continue exploring on your own. My experience has taught me that emotions and thoughts are part of the terrain; they are not the sole features of the landscape. Emotions provide a provocative palette that colors the peaks and valleys of our lives. They are tints and shades, not the mountain. Thoughts arise from the landscape, provide discourse on the journey, and attempt to divine what lies ahead. Thoughts direct us to the mountain, but they cannot become the mountain.

The greatest secret of all:

Simply thinking about your health goals will not bring them to fruition. In contrast, directed, effective action greatly improves your chances of creating health.

Action creates momentum that can move you toward your desired destination.

During a period of self-doubt and disillusionment, a beloved friend challenged me to make a decision and then act on it. "But I'm afraid I won't make the right decision," I whined.

"It really doesn't matter what you decide," he told me. "Just decide something. Get moving, get the wheels turning. God can't steer a parked truck!"

Even then, steeped as I was in misery, I laughed. I would offer you the same advice. Decide what is important to you. Determine whether or not you want to act on those desires. Remember, having a desire or a vision does not mean you are obligated to fulfill it. If you do want to create what matters most to you, take a deep breath, hold on to your hat, and take that first step. Continue stepping, evaluating and adjusting your actions as you move forward. You are embarking on the journey of a lifetime!

What this means for you:

The journey of a thousand miles begins with a single step. Create a vision of health, reconnoiter where you are, decide, and then **take action.**

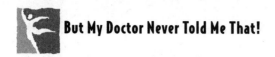 **But My Doctor Never Told Me That!**

N O T E S :

Appendix A:
Reviewing the Journey, Evaluating Your Progress

As you continue your journey to lifelong health, make dates with yourself to review your progress and re-evaluate your future course. Every traveler knows that journeys require constant adjustments – many factors will shape the journey to health. Astronauts traveling to the moon reported they were off course over 90 percent of the time! Our earth-bound ramblings need as much careful adjustment as an astronaut's lunar trajectory.

Once you have created your health destination, taken stock of your current location, and begun the steps toward health, I suggest you return to this section at regular intervals to re-evaluate your journey:

In three months:
1. Review Your Journey to Health
a. Health destination
- Revisit my life goals. Are the things I have envisioned still important to me?
- Do I need to be healthy in order to fulfill my life goals?
- Revisit my vision of health and ask, "Is this still where I want to go?"
- Have I already completed some of my initial goals?
- Add or subtract elements as needed.

b. Current location
- How close am I to my vision of health?
- What steps have I taken since I first developed my vision of health?
- How has my body responded?

- What measurements am I using to judge my response?
- How accurately am I measuring my progress?
- Review the exercise journal, diet diary, and exercise questionnaire from Chapter 3.
- What does my diet look like now?
- Has my exercise program changed?
- How am I supporting my mental and emotional health?

c. Notice the difference between where you are and where you want to be.

d. Simultaneously hold an image of your desired state and your current state of health. Notice the structural tension generated by the disparity between the two pictures.

e. Ask yourself, "If I could have my desired state of health, would I take it?"

f. If the answer is "Yes," then CHOOSE that state of health. "I choose . . ." and describe what you desire.

g. Fill in action steps that will move you toward your destination.

Action Steps to Health
- What steps will I take on my continued journey to health?
- Are the measurements appropriate to the goal?
- Which steps have been effective so far?
- Which actions have failed to move me forward or diverted me on my journey?
- What steps will move me closer to my vision?

2. **Meet With Your Support Group**

   If you have been working through the book with a
   group of friends, schedule a time to review your
   progress, discuss your challenges, and share
   your success.

In six months:

1. Reflect on your life vision – what do you want to
   create in your life?
2. Review your Journey to Health (see above).
3. Meet with your support group.
4. Repeat *The Stress Map* (see Appendix B for
   ordering information).

In 12 months:

1. Reflect on your life vision – what do you want to
   create in your life?
2. Review your Journey to Health (see above).
3. Meet with your support group.
4. Repeat *The Stress Map*.
5. See your physician for a complete annual exam.
   Physical exam:
   Blood work: Complete Blood Count, chemistry
   screen, thyroid function panel, cardiovascular test
   (e.g. treadmill), if applicable EKG (if above 50 years
   old, men and women), occult blood test, body
   composition test.
   Men:
   Prostate exam
   Testicular and penile exam
   Women:
   Pap smear
   Breast exam
   Mammogram (if applicable)
   DEXA bone mineral density scan (if applicable)

Appendix B
Resources by Chapter

Chapter 1: Dale's Story
For more information about the High Level
Wellness Program© or for personal consultations
with Dr. Judith Boice:
E-mail: drjudith@drjudithboice.com
Website: http//:www.drjudithboice.com
Telephone and Fax: (503) 252-9163

Chapter 2: Secrets for Optimizing Health
Plant Savers United
PO Box 98
East Barre, VT 05649
Telephone: (802) 479-9825
Fax: (802) 476-3722

Sharol Tilgner, N.D.
Wise Woman Herbals™, Inc.
PO Box 279
Creswell, Oregon 97426
Telephone: (541) 895-5152

Chapter 3: The Oracle of Hygieia
Order *The Stress Map* at your local
bookstore or directly from:
Newmarket Press
18 East 48th St.
 New York, NY 10017
Telephone: (212) 832-3575

Chapter 4: Secrets for Nourishing Your Body

Johanna Budwig, M.D. *Flax Oil as a True Aid for Arthritis, Heart Infarction, Cancer & Other Diseases.* Richmond, British Columbia: Apple Publishing Company Ltd., 1994.

Vita-Mix juicers, for juicing whole fruits and vegetables.
Vita-Mix Total Nutrition Center
8615 Usher Rd.
Cleveland, Ohio 44138
Telephone: 800-848-2348

Chapter 5: Classified Information About Exercise

- Bob Anderson. *Stretching.* Bolinas, CA: Shelter Publications, Inc., 1980.
- Covert Bailey. *The New Fit or Fat.* Boston, MA: Houghton Mifflin Co., 1991.
- Covert Bailey. *Smart Exercise: Burning Fat, Getting Fit.* Boston, MA: Houghton, Mifflin Co., 1996.
- The Firm workouts combine aerobics and strength training. Each tape begins with a warm up and ends with stretching.

Telephone: 800-THE-FIRM
FAX: 803-881-6583
Mail: The Firm
1007 Johnnie Dodds Blvd.
Mt. Pleasant, SC 29464-9934

Chapter 6: Secrets Your Doctor Never Told You About Mental and Emotional Health

- Joe Dominguez and Vicki Robin. *Your Money Or Your Life*. New York: Penguin Books, 1992.
- Robert Fritz. *Creating*. New York: Fawcett Columbine, 1991.
- Robert Fritz. *The Path of Least Resistance*. New York: Fawcett Columbine, 1989.
- James Maas, Ph.D. *Power Sleep*. New York: Random House, 1998.

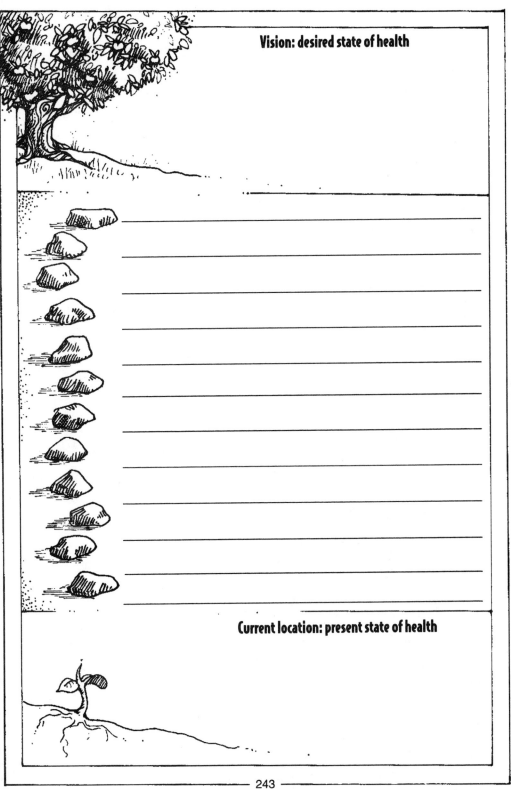

Vision: desired state of health

Current location: present state of health

DIET JOURNAL for _____   **Beginning Date** _____

The purpose of this diary is to provide you and your doctor with an unbiased record of your normal eating habits. Simply eat your typical diet and record what you eat for seven days in sucession. Under breakfast, lunch, and dinner columns list food and drink ingredients and amounts. Under BM, list bowel movement times. Under Notes, list symptoms such as mood swings, indigestion, headaches, fatigue, etc. Remember to include snacks.

Include supplements (brand name, ingredients, potency):

Breakfast DAY 1	Lunch	Dinner	BM Times	Notes
DAY 2				
DAY 3				

Breakfast	Lunch	Dinner	BM Times	Notes
DAY 4				
DAY 5				
DAY 6				
DAY 7				

Additional Notes _____

EXERCISE JOURNAL for _____   Beginning Date _____

The purpose of this diary is to provide you and your doctor with an unbiased record of your normal exercise habits. Simply follow your typical exercise routine and record what you do for seven days in sucession. For every day list the amount and type of exercise you do using the following descriptions. **Aerobic exercise (AE):** rhythmic, continuous exercise using the large muscles of the body (legs) that deepens breathing and increases the heart beat to target heart rate. Examples: walking, jogging, running, swimming, rowing. **Strength-building exercise (SBE):** resistance exercise that increases muscle strength. Examples: isometrics, calisthenics, weight lifting, sprinting. **Stretching exercise (SE):** stretching and holding muscles at just less than the point of discomfort. Examples: yoga. **Activities of Daily Living (ADL):** activities at work or at home that require movement, e.g. typing, vacuuming, gardening, driving, doing laundry.

	Responses to exercise. (Muscle strains after certain kinds of exercise, enjoyment or dislike of particular types of exercise, etc.)		
DAY I (AE) – (SBE) – (SE) – (ADL) –			
DAY 2			
DAY 3			

DAY 4 (AE) – (SBE) – (SE) – (ADL) –	
DAY 5	
DAY 6	
DAY 7	

Additional Notes _____

Exercise Adherence Questionnaire

This series of questions is intended to help you discover your attitudes, prejudices, and preferences about exercise. The questions are fuel for thought to help you discover the type of exercise that best suits you. *Directions: Check each statement that applies to you.*

Beliefs

——I am too old to exercise.

—— Exercise only helps if you do a lot, and I'm not an iron man!

——I think I am uncoordinated and feel too embarrassed to exercise.

——Exercise is all work and no play.

——I will be injured if I begin to exercise.

——Sweating is disgusting.

——Exercise is good for my health.

My Style

——I drive myself hard.

—— If something seems too hard, I will give up.

When I relapse from my exercise program due to injury or illness:

—— I probably won't start again.

—— I will ridicule myself for stopping my exercise program.

—— I will certainly begin exercising again.

——I prefer to exercise alone.

——I love team sports.

——I would exercise more consistently if I worked out with a group or a friend.

——I want immediate results or I will not stick to my program.

Exercise Adherence Questionnaire

My Support Team

____The people I live with think exercise is silly.

____Even though no one at home supports my exercise program, I have a friend or family member who will.

____The people I live with will be neutral about my exercise program.

____The people I live with will be encouraging of my exercise program.

____I care what other people think of me.

____I don't give a hoot about what others think.

My choices

____I have chosen to exercise to support my vision of health.

____I can't exercise now . . . . maybe later.

____Not now, not ever!

My History

____I was usually the last one picked for school teams.

____I have been made fun of playing sports or wearing a bathing suit.

____I was a super jock in high school or college.

____Moderate exercise has always been part of my daily life.

Endnotes by chapter

Chapter 2: Secrets for Optimizing Health

[1] Andreoli, T.E. et al. *Cecil: Essentials of Medicine.* Philadelphia: Harcourt Brace Jovanovich, 1990, 63.

[2] Ornish, D.M. et al. "Can lifestyle changes reverse coronary heart disease? The Lifestyle Heart Trial," *Lancet* 336, no. 8708 (July 1990): 129-33.

[3] Lazarou, J.; B.H. Pomeranz; P.N. Corey. "Incidents of adverse drug reactions in hospitalized patients: a meta-analysis of prospective studies," *JAMA* 270, no. 15 (April 15, 1998): 1200-5.

[4] Moss, Richard. *How Shall I Live.* Berkeley, CA: Celestial Arts, 1985, 45.

Chapter 4: Secrets for Nourishing Your Body

[1] Worthington, V. "Effect of agricultural methods on nutritional quality: a comparison of organic with conventional crops," *Altern Ther Health Med* 4, no. 1 (January 1998): 58-69.

[2] Sherman, H.C. "Calcium requirements of maintenance in man," *J Biol Chem* 44 (1920): 21-27.

[3] Heaney, R.P. "Cofactors influencing the calcium requirement – other nutrients." Paper presented at the NIH Consensus Development Conference on Optimal Calcium Intake, Bethesda, MD, June 1994.

[4] Hegsted, M. et al. "Urinary calcium and calcium balance in young men as affected by level of protein and phosphorus intake," *J Nutr* 111 (1981): 553-562.

5 Budwig, Johanna. *Flax Oil as a True Aid Against Arthritis, Heart Infarction, Cancer, and Other Diseases*. Vancouver, BC: Apple Publishing Company, Ltd, 1992 & 1994, 7.

6 Burr, M.L. et al. "Effects of changes in fat, fish, and fibre intakes on death and myocardial reinfarction: diet and reinfarction trial (DART)," *Lancet* 2, no. 8666 (September 30, 1998): 757-761.

7 Willet, W.C. et al. "Intake of *trans* fatty acids and risk of coronary heart disease among women," *Lancet* 69 (1993): 3-19.

8 De Lorgeril, M. et al. "Control of bias in dietary trial to prevent coronary recurrences: the Lyon diet heart study," *Eur J Clin Nutr* 51 (1997): 116-122.

Chapter 5: Classified Information About Exercise

1 Seals, D.R. et al. "Effect of regular aerobic exercise on elevated blood pressure in postmenopausal women," *Am J Cardiol* 80, no. 1 (July 1997): 49-55.

2 Pedersen, B.K. "Influence of physical activity on the cellular immune system: mechanisms of action," *Int J Sports Med* 12 (June 1991), suppl 1: S23-9.

3 Rodriguez, A.B. et al. "Phagocytic function of blood neutrophils in sedentary young people after physical exercise," *Int J Sports Med* 12, no. 3 (June 1991): 276-80.

4 Smith, J.A. et al. "Exercise, training and neutrophil microbicidal activity," *Int J Sports Med* 11, no. 3 (June 1990): 179-87.

5 Henderson, N.K.; C.P. White; J.A. Eisman. "The roles of exercise and fall risk reduction in the prevention of osteoporosis," *Endocrinol Metab Clin North Am* 27, no. 2 (June 1998): 369-387.

6 Stillman, R.J. et al. "Physical activity and bone mineral content in women aged 30 to 85 years," *Med Sci Sports Exerc* 18, no. 5 (October 1986): 576-580.

7 Sinaki, M. and K.P. Offord. "Physical activity in post-menopausal women: effect on back muscle strength and bone mineral density of the spine," *Arch Phys Med Rehabil* 69, no. 4 (April 1988): 277-280.

8 Jakicic, J.M. et al. "Prescribing exercise in multiple short bouts versus one continuous bout: effects on adherence, cardiorespiratory fitness, and weight loss in overweight women," *Int J Obes Relat Metab Disord* 19, no. 12 (December 1995): 893-901.

9 Fiatarone, M.A. et al. "Exercise training and nutritional supplementation for physical frailty in very elderly people," *N Engl J Med* 330, no. 25 (June 1994): 1769-75.

10 Kase, Lori Miller. "Lift weight to lose it," *Vogue* 181, no. 4 (April 1991): 222(2).

Chapter 6: Secrets Your Doctor Never Told You About Mental and Emotional Health

1 Fritz, Robert. *Creating.* New York: Ballantine Books, 1991, 123.

2 Ibid., 19-20.

3 Seals, D.R. et al. "Effect of regular aerobic exercise on elevated blood pressure in postmenopausal women," *American Journal of Cardiology* 80, no. 1 (July 1997): 49-55.

4 Barefoot, J.C. et al. "Depression and long-term mortality risk in patients with coronary artery disease," *American Journal of Cardiology* 78, no. 6 (September 15 1996): 613-17.

5 Vein, A.M. et al. "Physical exercise and nocturnal sleep in healthy humans," *Human Physiology* 17 (1991): 391-397.

6 Krueger, J.M. and J.A. Majde. "Sleep as a host defense: its regulation by microbial products and cytokines," *Clinical Immunology and Immunopathology* (1990): 188-199.

7 Irwin, Michael et al. *Journal of the Federation of American Societies for Experimental Biology* 10 (1996): 643-653.

8 Smith, Carlyel and Lorelei Lapp. "Increases in number of REMS and REM density in humans following an intensive learning period," *Sleep* 14 (1991): 325-330.

9 Dujardin, Kathy et al. "Sleep, brain activation, and cognition," *Physiology and Behavior* 47 (1990): 1271-1278.

10 Mass, James. *Power Sleep*. New York: Random House, 1998, 72-73.

11 Dominguez, Joe and Vicki Robin. *Your Money Or Your Life*. New York: Penguin Books, 1992, 112.

12 Ibid., 116-117.

About the author

Dr. Judith Boice, author, international teacher, Naturopathic physician and acupuncturist, has a special passion for working with wellness and women's health. Dr. Boice created "The High Level Wellness Program©" to support individuals in achieving their personal life and health goals. She designed the Wellness Program for patients who wanted to improve their health but were unsure of where or how to begin.

Other creative passions include photography, music, and gardening. Her photographs have appeared in several magazines and newspapers, *Trees for Life* calendars, and Sierra Club Books publications.

Dr. Boice is the author of several magazine articles and five books, including *The Pocket Guide to Naturopathic Medicine*. A Phi Beta Kappa graduate of Oberlin College, she has lived and traveled around the world, fostering an understanding and respect for many cultures and traditions.

BOOKS BY DR. JUDITH BOICE

The Pocket Guide to Naturopathic Medicine, Crossing Press, 1996. This small, pocket-sized volume is perfect for a first aid kit at home or on the road.

The Mother Earth Postcard Book, Sierra Club Books, 1993. This collection features 20 stunning images by women nature photographers.

The Art of Daily Activism, Wingbow Press, 1992. "Judith Boice has created an engaging guide for moving from apathy to awareness to activism. I hope her advice and encouragement will be taken to heart." Charlene Spretnak, co-author of *Green Politics.*

At One With All Life: A Personal Journey in Gaian Communities, Findhorn Press, 1990. Follow the author on a journey that spans four communities on four continents: the Bear Tribe in Washington state, the Findhorn Foundation in Scotland, Auroville in India, and a traditional aboriginal settlement in Australia's Western Desert.

AUDIO CASSETTES:

Make No Bones About It: Straight Talk on Preventing and Treating Osteoporosis. Discover how diet, exercise, supplements, drugs, and hormones affect bone health. Learn how to build strong bones, no matter what your age.

Menopause: Naturally. Dr. Boice discusses lifestyle factors, phytoestrogens, and natural hormones that can ease the passage through menopause.

(see next page for ordering information)

Order Form

for books and tapes
by Dr. Judith Boice

Books	Cost	x	Quantity	=	TOTAL
The Pocket Guide to Naturopathic Medicine	$6.95 ea.				$
The Mother Earth Postcard Book	$9.00 ea.				$
The Art of Daily Activism	$13.95 ea.				$
At One With All Life	$14.95 ea.				$
Audio Cassettes					
Make No Bones About It	$9.00 ea.				$
Menopause: Naturally	$9.00 ea.				$
Video Cassette					
Menopause: Naturally	$19.95 ea.				$

SUBTOTAL $ _____

Please allow
four to six weeks
for delivery.

Shipping and handling   + $ __5.00__
(First book or tape $5.00)

Each additional item add $2.00   +   _____

ORDER TOTAL $ _____
(Sales tax not required for items purchased in Oregon)

SHIP TO:_____

ADDRESS: _____

CITY: _____STATE: _____ZIP: _____

PHONE: (day)_____ (evening) _____

Please copy order form, enclose, and include a check payable to: Dr. Judith Boice.

Mail to: ALTHEA PRESS 11520 SE Main St. Portland, OR 97216

Thank you for your order!